D0223631

Emergency and Acute Medicine
on the move

Emergency and Acute Medicine
on the move

Authors: Naomi Meardon,
Shireen Siddiqui and Elena Del Vescovo
Editors: Lucy C. Peart and Sherif Hemaya
Editorial Advisor: Alan Fletcher

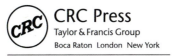

CRC Press
Taylor & Francis Group
Boca Raton London New York

CRC Press is an imprint of the
Taylor & Francis Group, an **informa** business

CRC Press
Taylor & Francis Group
6000 Broken Sound Parkway NW, Suite 300
Boca Raton, FL 33487-2742

© 2016 by Naomi Meardon,Shireen Siddiqui,Elena Del Vescovo
CRC Press is an imprint of Taylor & Francis Group, an Informa business

No claim to original U.S. Government works

Printed on acid-free paper
Version Date: 20150617

International Standard Book Number-13: 978-1-4441-4569-4 (Pack - Book and Ebook)

Contents

Preface

Have you ever found emergency and acute medicine bland or overwhelmingly complicated? Do you often forget the basics or struggle with the core texts? Are you simply short of time and have exams looming? If so, then this short revision guide will help you. Written by students for students, this book presents information in a wide range of forms including flow charts, colourful diagrams and summary tables. No matter what your learning style, we think you will find this book appealing and easy to read. Its innovative style will help you, the reader, to connect with this often-feared topic – helping you to learn and understand it, and maybe even enjoy it, while also helping to bridge the gap to the recommended core texts.

AUTHORS

Naomi Meardon BMedSci (Hons) MBChB – Core Trainee Year 1 in Medicine, Chesterfield Royal Hospital, UK

Shireen Siddiqui MBChB MRCGP DFSRH DRCOG – General Practitioner, London, UK

Elena Del Vescovo BMedSci (Hons) MBChB – Speciality Trainee Year 2 in Radiology, Royal Infirmary of Edinburgh, NHS Lothian, UK

EDITORS

Lucy C Peart BSc MBChB MRCP PgDip – Speciality Registrar Acute Medicine, Sheffield Teaching Hospitals, Sheffield, UK

Sherif Hemaya MB BCh FCEM – Emergency Medicine Consultant, Northern General Hospital, Sheffield Teaching Hospitals NHS Foundation Trust, Sheffield, UK

EDITORIAL ADVISOR

Alan Fletcher BMedSci (Hons) MBChB MRCPath (Affiliate) FRCP (Edin) FCEM – Consultant in Emergency Medicine and Acute Medicine, Sheffield Teaching Hospitals NHS Foundation Trust, Sheffield, UK

EDITOR-IN-CHIEF

Rory Mackinnon BSc (Hons) MBChB – GP Registrar, Oxford Terrace & Rawling Road Medical Group, Gateshead, UK

SERIES EDITORS

Sally Keat BMedSci MBChB – Foundation Year 2 doctor, Northern General Hospital, Sheffield, UK

Thomas Locke BSc MBChB – Foundation Year 2 doctor, Northern General Hospital, Sheffield, UK
Andrew Walker BMedSci MBChB MRCP (UK) – Speciality Trainee Year 2 in Medicine, Northern General Hospital, Sheffield, UK

Acknowledgements

The authors thank everyone who has contributed their expertise in order to bring this book to print.

Reference values

FULL BLOOD COUNT

Haemoglobin (Hb)	11–14.7 g/dL (females), 13.1–16.6 g/dL (males)
White cell count (WCC)	$3.5–9.5 \times 10^9$/L
Platelets (Plt)	$140–370 \times 10^9$/L
Haematocrit (HCT)	0.32–0.43 L/L (females), 0.38–0.48 L/L (males)
Mean cell volume (MCV)	80.0–98.1 fL (females), 81.8–96.3 fL (males)
Mean cell haemoglobin (MCH)	27.0–34.2 pg
Mean cell haemoglobin concentration (MCHC)	33.5–35.5 g/dL
Neutrophils	$1.7–6.5 \times 10^9$/L
Lymphocytes	$1.0–3.0 \times 10^9$/L
Monocytes	$0.25–1.0 \times 10^9$/L
Eosinophils	$0.04–0.5 \times 10^9$/L
Basophils	$0–0.1 \times 10^9$/L

IRON PROFILE

Iron	8–33	μmol/L
% IBC saturation	20–50	%
Total iron binding capacity (TIBC)	45–81	μmol/L
Ferritin	30–400	ng/mL

B_{12} AND FOLATE

B_{12}	211–911 ng/L
Folate – Deficient <3.4 μg/L Borderline 3.4–5.3 μg/L	

CLOTTING

PT	9.5–11.5 s
APTT	25.5–37.5 s
Fibrinogen	1.4–3.5 g/L

U&E

Sodium	134–143 mmol/L
Potassium	3.6–5.3 mmol/L
Urea	2.3–7.7 mmol/L
Creatinine	66–118 µmol/L
Bicarbonate	22–32 mmol/L
Chloride	95–107 mmol/L
Magnesium	0.7–1.0 mmol/L
Creatine kinase	34–306 IU/L

OSMOLALITIES

Urine sodium	Normal <20 mmol/L
Urine osmolality	Normal <500 mOsm/kg H_2O
Serum osmolality	280–295 mOsm/kg H_2O

LFTS

Total protein	63–79	g/L
Albumin	35–48	g/L
Globulin	18–36	g/L
Total bilirubin	5–28	µmol/L
Alkaline phosphatase	36–125	IU/L
AST	15–41	IU/L
ALT	17–63	IU/L
GGT	7–50	IU/L

TFTS

TSH	0.35–4.5 mIU/L
FT_3	3.5–6.5 pmol/L
FT_4	10.0–19.8 pmol/L

CALCIUM & PHOSPHATE

Corrected calcium	2.2–2.6 mmol/L
Phosphate	0.8–1.5 mmol/L

SERUM CORTISOL

Normal range	a.m., 198–720 nmol/L; p.m., 85–459 nmol/L

ABG

pH	7.35–7.45
PaO_2	11–13 kPa
$PaCO_2$	4.7–6.0 kPa
HCO_3^-	22–28 mmol/L
Base excess	−2 to +2 mmol/L
Anion gap	12–16 mmol/L

LIPID PROFILE

Cholesterol	Target in patients with ischaemic heart disease is <5.0 mmol/L
Triglycerides	Elevated if >2.0 mmol/L

HDL CHOLESTEROL

High risk	Male, <1.0 mmol/L; Female, <1.1 mmol/L

List of abbreviations

- AAA: Abdominal aortic aneurysm
- ABCDE: Airway, breathing, circulation, disability, exposure
- ABG: Arterial blood gas
- Abx: Antibiotics
- ACE inhibitor: Angiotensin-converting enzyme inhibitor
- ACL: Anterior cruciate ligament
- ACS: Acute coronary syndrome
- AF: Atrial fibrillation
- AP: Antero-posterior
- ARF: Acute renal failure
- AXR: Abdominal X-ray
- BD: Twice daily
- BM: Blood glucose level
- BNF: British national formulary
- BP: Blood pressure
- C-spine: Cervical spine
- CK: Creatinine kinase
- COPD: Chronic obstructive pulmonary disease
- CPR: Cardiopulmonary resuscitation
- CRP: C-reactive protein
- CRT: Capillary refill time
- CSF: Cerebrospinal fluid
- CVA: Cerebrovascular accident
- CVP: Central venous pressure
- CXR: Chest X-ray
- DIC: Disseminated intravascular coagulation
- DKA: Diabetic ketoacidosis
- DVT: Deep vein thrombosis
- ECG: Electrocardiogram
- ECT: Electroconvulsive therapy
- ESR: Erythrocyte sedimentation rate
- FBC: Full blood count
- FFP: Fresh frozen plasma
- G+S: Group and save
- GCS: Glasgow Coma Scale
- GTN: Glyceryl trinitrate
- Hb: Haemoglobin
- HB: Heart block
- HDU: High dependency unit

- HELLP: Haemolysis, elevated liver tests, low platelets
- HHS: Hyperglycaemic hyperosmolar state
- HONK: See HHS
- HR: Heart rate
- IBD: Inflammatory bowel disease
- IBS: Irritable bowel syndrome
- ICU: Intensive care unit
- ID: Infectious diseases
- IM: Intramuscular
- IV: Intravenous
- IVU: Intravenous urogram
- JVP: Jugular venous pressure
- K^+: Potassium
- KUB: Kidneys, ureter, bladder
- LBBB: Left bundle branch block
- LFT: Liver function test
- LMN: Lower motor neurone
- LMP: Last menstrual period
- LP: Lumbar puncture
- LRTI: Lower respiratory tract infection
- LVH: Left ventricular hypertrophy
- MC&S: Microscopy, culture and sensitivity
- MI: Myocardial infarction
- MMSE: Mini mental state examination
- Na^+: Sodium
- NBM: Nil by mouth
- NIV: Non-invasive ventilation
- NSAID: Non-steroidal anti-inflammatory drug
- NSTEMI: Non-ST elevation myocardial infarction
- OD: Once daily
- OGD: Oesophogastroduodenoscopy
- PCI: Percutaneous coronary intervention
- PO: Oral
- PPI: Proton pump inhibitor
- PR: Per rectum
- PTT: Prothrombin time
- QDS: Four times daily
- RR: Respiratory rate
- RTA: Road traffic accident
- RUQ: Right upper quadrant
- SOB: Shortness of breath
- SpO_2: Oxygen saturation
- STEMI: ST elevation myocardial infarction

- STI: Sexually transmitted infection
- TCA: Tricyclic antidepressant
- TDS: Three times daily
- TFT: Thyroid function test
- U&E: Urea and electrolyte
- UA: Unstable angina
- UC: Ulcerative colitis
- UMN: Upper motor neurone
- UO: Urine output
- URTI: Upper respiratory tract infection
- UTI: Urinary tract infection
- VF: Ventricular fibrillation
- VT: Ventricular tachycardia
- WCC: White cell count

An explanation of the text

The book is divided into two parts: emergency and acute medicine, and a self-assessment section. We have used bullet points to keep the text concise and supplemented this with a range of diagrams, pictures and MICRO-boxes (explained below).

Where possible, we have endeavoured to include treatment options for the conditions covered. Nevertheless, drug sensitivities and clinical practices are constantly under review, so always check your local guidelines for up-to-date information.

MICRO-facts

These boxes expand on the text and contain clinically relevant facts and memorable summaries of the essential information.

MICRO-print

These boxes contain additional information to the text that may interest certain readers but is not essential for everybody to learn.

MICRO-case

These boxes contain clinical cases relevant to the text and include a number of summary bullet points to highlight the key learning objectives.

MICRO-reference

These boxes contain references to important clinical research and national guidance.

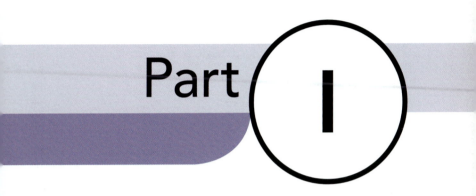

Part I

Emergency and acute medicine

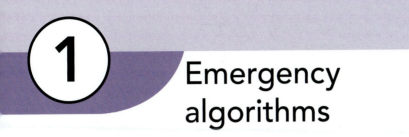

1 Emergency algorithms

1.1 ASSESSING THE ACUTELY UNWELL PATIENT

The ABCDE approach

- An acute assessment algorithm which stands for:
    - Airway
    - Breathing
    - Circulation
    - Disability
    - Exposure
- Used to systematically evaluate a patient's condition in order of importance of life-threatening pathologies.

Procedure

- See Fig. 1.1.
- Start by assessing the airway.
- Once airway stable, move on to breathing.
- Return to 'A' if the patient becomes unstable or a treatment or procedure has been performed.
- Continue through ABCDE in this fashion until the patient is stable.
- It is vital to re-assess regularly to evaluate the effects of treatment.

Airway

Assessment:
- Inspect the airway.
- Remove any obvious foreign body from the mouth or oropharynx under direct vision using McGill's forceps or suction to remove vomit or secretions.
- Listen to the airway for sounds of obstruction; stridor/snoring/gurgling.

Management:
- Jaw-thrust/head-tilt/chin-lift (cervical spine control in trauma).
- Airway adjuncts: oropharyngeal/nasopharyngeal airways (beware of basal skull fracture).
- Intubation/Laryngeal mask airway: consider if airway still compromised.

Breathing

Assessment:
- Look for chest expansion/fogging of oxygen mask/cyanosis/breathing pattern.
- Feel for chest expansion (equal bilaterally or reduced)?
- Feel for position of trachea (midline or deviated)?
- Percuss the chest (resonant or dull)?
- Auscultate the chest for air entry (equal bilaterally or reduced)?
- Possibility of tension pneumothorax? Reduced air entry with hyper-resonance and decreased expansion on affected side with tracheal deviation away and distended neck veins.

Management:
- High flow O_2: 15L/min via a non-rebreathe mask.
- Bag valve mask (BVM): poor respiratory effort or apnoea.

Monitor:
- SpO_2, RR, PEFR (if able), capnography.

Circulation

Assessment:
- Look for pallor, signs of bleeding, mottling, vasodilatation/constriction.
- Feel central pulses and peripheral pulses – carotid/femoral (rate/rhythm/volume/character).
- Capillary refill (>2 seconds abnormal).
- Signs of AAA and DVT.

Management:
- Secure IV access.
- Take bloods including FBC, G+S or X-match, full profile, clotting screen, cardiac markers if applicable.
- Consider IV fluid challenge if shocked.

Monitor:
- Cardiac monitor.
- Attach and monitor via defibrillator if peri-arrest.
- HR, NIBP/IBP monitoring/urine output monitoring via urinary catheter.
- 12 lead ECG.

Disability

Assessment:
- AVPU/GCS.
- Pupillary/plantar reflexes/CNS and PNS examination.
- Check blood glucose.

Exposure

Assessment:
- Remove all clothing.
- Check temperature.
- Check for rashes/wounds.

Management:
- Cover patient with blankets to maintain normothermia.
- Consider rewarming techniques if hypothermic: forced air warming blankets, warm IV fluids, humidified O_2.

Fig. 1.1 Assessing the unwell patient ABCDE algorithm.

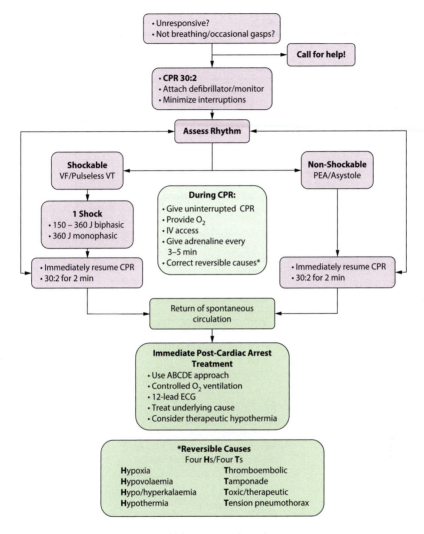

Fig. 1.2 Cardiac arrest/advanced life support algorithm.

1.2 ANAPHYLAXIS

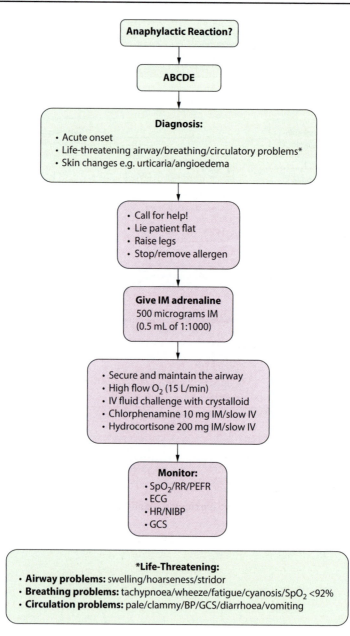

Anaphylactic Reaction?

ABCDE

Diagnosis:
- Acute onset
- Life-threatening airway/breathing/circulatory problems*
- Skin changes e.g. urticaria/angioedema

- Call for help!
- Lie patient flat
- Raise legs
- Stop/remove allergen

Give IM adrenaline
500 micrograms IM
(0.5 mL of 1:1000)

- Secure and maintain the airway
- High flow O_2 (15 L/min)
- IV fluid challenge with crystalloid
- Chlorphenamine 10 mg IM/slow IV
- Hydrocortisone 200 mg IM/slow IV

Monitor:
- SpO$_2$/RR/PEFR
- ECG
- HR/NIBP
- GCS

*Life-Threatening:
- **Airway problems:** swelling/hoarseness/stridor
- **Breathing problems:** tachypnoea/wheeze/fatigue/cyanosis/SpO$_2$ <92%
- **Circulation problems:** pale/clammy/BP/GCS/diarrhoea/vomiting

Fig. 1.3 Management of anaphylaxis algorithm.

Emergency and acute medicine

1.3 ANALGESIA

Methods of pain relief
- Analgesia (see Fig. 1.4)
- Injury-specific relief:
  - Reduction/immobilization of fractures
  - GTN/O_2 in cardiac chest pain

Analgesic drugs
- Should be prescribed according to severity of pain as follows:
  - Prescribe the lowest dose required to relieve pain.
  - Titrate dose/change drug as required.
  - Choose drugs with the lowest possible side-effect profile.
  - Consider side-effect management with additional therapies.

Specific drug considerations
- Paracetamol:
  - Low side-effect profile
  - Anti-pyretic
  - Overdosage may lead to liver damage (see Section 10)
- Aspirin:
  - Anti-inflammatory properties
  - Increased bleeding risk
  - May exacerbate asthma
  - May cause gastric irritation
  - Consider adding proton pump inhibitor, e.g. omeprazole 20 mg once daily, orally
- NSAIDs, e.g. ibuprofen/diclofenac:
  - Anti-inflammatory properties
  - May cause gastric irritation
  - Consider PPI (as above)
  - May precipitate renal failure
  - May exacerbate asthma
  - Avoid in the elderly as high risk of renal impairment and GI bleeding
- Opioids:
  - Weak opioids may be given orally for chronic moderate pain
  - Strong opioids may be given IV in acute conditions
  - May cause nausea: add anti-emetic, e.g. cyclizine 50 mg IM
  - May cause constipation: add PRN laxative, e.g. lactulose

Emergency and acute medicine

Analgesic ladder prescription algorithm

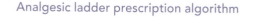

Step 1: Mild Pain
- **1st Line** = Paracetamol 1g QDS PO
- **2nd Line** = NSAIDs (1st line if predominantly inflammatory)
  - Ibuprofen 200–400 mg TDS PO (mild pain)
  - Diclofenac 50 mg TDS PO (moderate pain)

↓

Step 2: Moderate Pain
- Add low dose weak opioid e.g. codeine 30–60 mg QDS PO
- Weak opioid alone e.g. dihydrocodeine 30 QDS PO

↓

Step 3: Moderate–Severe Pain
- **High dose weak opioid:**
  - Dihydrocodeine 60 mg QDS PO
  - Tramadol 50–100 mg QDS

↓

Step 4: Severe Pain
- **Strong opioid:**
  - Acute → Morphine IV 2.5–10 mg depending on patient weight/severity of pain
  - Chronic → Oramorph PO 5–10 mg 1–2 hrly

Fig. 1.4 Analgesia prescription algorithm.

2 Clinical presentations

Clinical presentation flowcharts

- This section is divided into various clinical presentations as a tool to enable you to review basic investigation and management plans.
- The sections of the flowchart are divided as follows:
  - Concerning features:
    - Any of these features in a patient requires urgent senior review.
  - Standard investigations:
    - These investigations should be performed on all patients with the named clinical presentation.
  - Further investigations:
    - These are additional investigations that may give more diagnostic information.
  - Differential diagnosis:
    - The various conditions that can present with the named clinical presentations are listed and briefly discussed here.
    - A page reference is given to the section in the book where a more detailed explanation is given.

KEY FEATURES

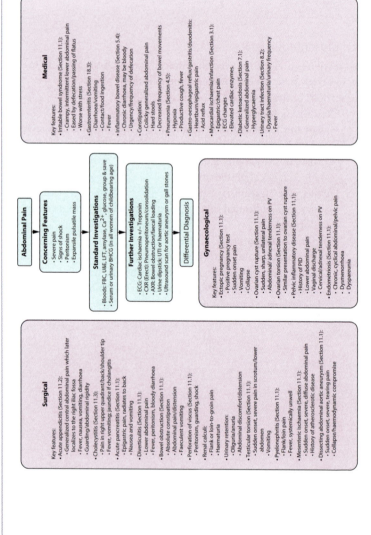

Abdominal Pain

Concerning Features
- Severe pain
- Signs of shock
- Peritonism
- Expansile pulsatile mass

Standard Investigations
- Bloods: FBC, U&E, LFT, amylase, Ca²⁺, glucose, group & save
- Serum or urinary BHCG (in all women of childbearing age)

Further Investigations
- ECG: Cardiac ischaemia +/- Troponin
- CXR (Erect): Pneumoperitoneum/consolidation
- AXR: Bowel obstruction/faecal loading
- Urine dipstick UTI or haematuria
- Ultrasound scan for aortic aneurysm or gall stones

Differential Diagnosis

Surgical

Key features:
- Acute appendicitis (Section 11.2):
  - Generalized central abdominal pain which later localizes to the right iliac fossa
  - Fever, nausea, vomiting, diarrhoea
  - Guarding/abdominal rigidity
- Cholecystitis (Section 11.3):
  - Pain in right upper quadrant/back/shoulder tip
  - Fever, vomiting; jaundice if cholangitis
- Acute pancreatitis (Section 11.1):
  - Epigastric pain, radiates to back
  - Nausea and vomiting
- Diverticulitis (Section 11.1):
  - Lower abdominal pain
  - Fever, peritonism, bloody diarrhoea
- Bowel obstruction (Section 11.1):
  - Absolute constipation
  - Abdominal pain/distension
  - Faeculent vomiting
- Perforation of viscus (Section 11.1):
  - Peritonism, guarding, shock
- Renal calculi:
  - Flank or loin-to-groin pain
  - Haematuria
- Urinary retention:
  - Oliguria/anuria
  - Abdominal discomfort/distension
- Testicular torsion (Section 11.1):
  - Sudden onset, severe pain in scrotum/lower abdomen
  - Vomiting
- Pyelonephritis (Section 11.1):
  - Flank/loin pain
  - Fever, systemically unwell
- Mesenteric ischaemia (Section 11.1):
  - Sudden onset, severe, diffuse abdominal pain
  - History of atherosclerotic disease
- Dissecting abdominal aortic aneurysm (Section 11.1):
  - Sudden onset, severe, tearing pain
  - Collapse/haemodynamic compromise

Gynaecological

Key features:
- Ectopic pregnancy (Section 11.1):
  - Positive pregnancy test
  - Sudden onset pain
  - Vomiting
  - Collapse
- Ovarian cyst rupture (Section 11.1):
  - Sudden, sharp, unilateral pain
  - Abdominal/ adnexal tenderness on PV
- Ovarian torsion (Section 11.1):
  - Similar presentation to ovarian cyst rupture
- Pelvic inflammatory disease (Section 11.1):
  - History of PID
  - Lower abdominal pain
  - Vaginal discharge
  - Cervical/adnexal tenderness on PV
- Endometriosis (Section 11.1):
  - Chronic, cyclical abdominal/pelvic pain
  - Dysmenorrhoea
  - Dyspareunia

Medical

Key features:
- Irritable bowel syndrome (Section 11.1):
  - Crampy, intermittent lower abdominal pain
  - Eased by defecation/passing of flatus
  - Worse with stress
- Gastroenteritis (Section 18.3):
  - Diarrhoea/vomiting
  - Contact/food ingestion
  - Fever
- Inflammatory bowel disease (Section 5.4):
  - Chronic diarrhoea, may be bloody
  - Urgency/frequency of defecation
- Constipation:
  - Colicky generalized abdominal pain
  - Hard stools
  - Decreased frequency of bowel movements
- Pneumonia (Section 4.5):
  - Hypoxia
  - Productive cough, fever
- Gastro-oesophageal reflux/gastritis/duodenitis:
  - Heartburn/epigastric pain
  - Acid reflux
- Myocardial ischaemia/infarction (Section 3.1):
  - Epigastric/chest pain
  - ECG changes
  - Elevated cardiac enzymes.
- Diabetic ketoacidosis (Section 7.1):
  - Generalized abdominal pain
  - Hyperglycaemia
- Urinary tract infection (Section 8.2):
  - Dysuria/haematuria/urinary frequency
  - Fever

Fig. 2.1 Abdominal pain.

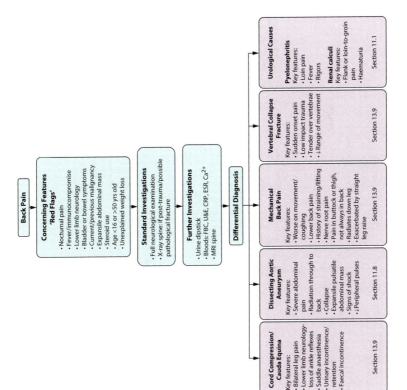

Fig. 2.2 Back pain.

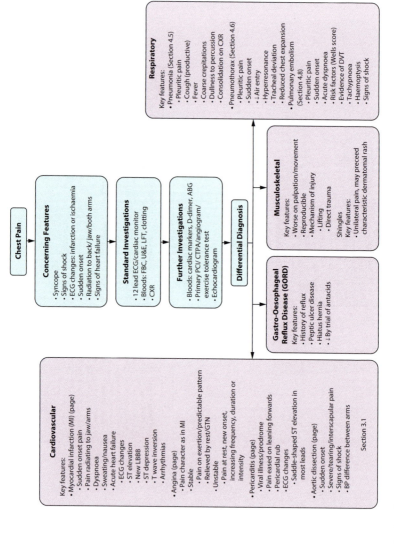

Chest Pain

Concerning Features
- Syncope
- Signs of shock
- ECG changes: infarction or ischaemia
- Sudden onset
- Radiation to back/jaw/both arms
- Signs of heart failure

Standard Investigations
- 12 lead ECG/cardiac monitor
- Bloods: FBC, U&E, LFT, clotting
- CXR

Further Investigations
- Bloods: cardiac markers, D-dimer, ABG
- Primary PCI/ CTPA/angiogram/ exercise tolerance test
- Echocardiogram

Differential Diagnosis

Respiratory
Key features:
- Pneumonia (Section 4.5)
  - Pleuritic pain
  - Cough (productive)
  - Fever
  - Coarse crepitations
  - Dullness to percussion
  - Consolidation on CXR
- Pneumothorax (Section 4.6)
  - Pleuritic pain
  - Sudden onset
  - ↓ Air entry
  - Hyperresonance
  - Tracheal deviation
  - Reduced chest expansion
- Pulmonary embolism (Section 4.8)
  - Pleuritic pain
  - Acute dyspnoea
  - Sudden onset
  - Risk factors (Wells score)
  - Evidence of DVT
  - Tachypnoea
  - Haemoptysis
  - Signs of shock

Musculoskeletal
Key features:
- Worse on palpation/movement
- Reproducible
- Mechanism of injury
  - Lifting
  - Direct trauma

Shingles
Key features:
- Unilateral pain, may preceed characteristic dermatomal rash

Gastro-Oesophageal Reflux Disease (GORD)
Key features:
- History of reflux
- Peptic ulcer disease
- Hiatus hernia
- ↓ By trial of antacids

Cardiovascular
Key features:
- Myocardial infarction (MI) (page)
  - Sudden onset pain
  - Pain radiating to jaw/arms
  - Dyspnoea
  - Sweating/nausea
  - Acute heart failure
  - ECG changes
    - ST elevation
    - New LBBB
    - ST depression
    - T wave inversion
  - Arrhythmias
- Angina (page)
  - Pain character as in MI
  - Stable
    - Pain on exertion/predictable pattern
    - Relieved by rest/GTN
  - Unstable
    - Pain at rest, new onset, increasing frequency, duration or intensity
- Pericarditis (page)
  - Viral illness/prodrome
  - Pain eased on leaning forwards
  - Pericardial rub
  - ECG changes
    - Saddle-shaped ST elevation in most leads
- Aortic dissection (page)
  - Sudden onset
  - Severe/tearing/interscapular pain
  - Signs of shock
  - BP difference between arms

Section 3.1

Fig. 2.3 Chest pain.

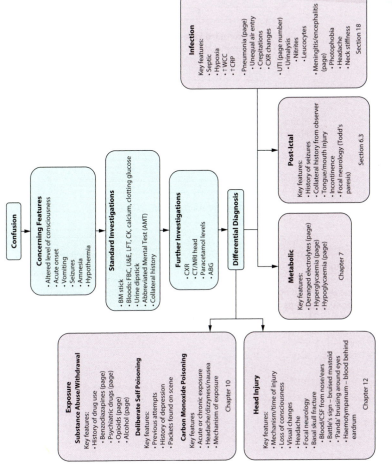

Confusion

Concerning Features
- Altered level of consciousness
- Acute onset
- Vomiting
- Seizures
- Amnesia
- Hypothermia

Standard Investigations
- BM stick
- Bloods: FBC, U&E, LFT, CK, calcium, clotting glucose
- Urine dipstick
- Abbreviated Mental Test (AMT)
- Collateral history

Further Investigations
- CXR
- CT/MRI head
- Paracetamol levels
- ABG

Differential Diagnosis

Infection
Key features:
- Septic
- Hypoxia
- ↑ WCC
- ↑ CRP
- Pneumonia (page)
- Unequal air entry
- Crepitations
- CXR changes
- UTI (page number)
- Urinalysis
  - Nitrites
  - Leucocytes
- Meningitis/encephalitis (page)
- Photophobia
- Headache
- Neck stiffness
Section 18

Post-Ictal
Key features:
- History of seizures
- Collateral history from observer
- Tongue/mouth injury
- Incontinence
- Focal neurology (Todd's paresis)
Section 6.3

Metabolic
Key features:
- Deranged electrolytes (page)
- Hyperglycaemia (page)
- Hypoglycaemia (page)
Chapter 7

Exposure
Substance Abuse/Withdrawal
Key features:
- History of drug use
  - Benzodiazapines (page)
  - Psychiatric drugs (page)
  - Opioids (page)
  - Alcohol (page)

Deliberate Self Poisoning
Key features:
- Previous attempts
- History of depression
- Packets found on scene

Carbon Monoxide Poisoning
Key features
- Acute or chronic exposure
- Headache/dizzyness/nausea
- Mechanism of exposure
Chapter 10

Head Injury
Key features:
- Mechanism/time of injury
- Loss of consciousness
- Visual changes
- Headache
- Focal neurology
- Basal skull fracture
  - Blood/CSF from nose/ears
  - Battle's sign – bruised mastoid
  - 'Panda' bruising around eyes
  - Haemotympanum – blood behind eardrum
Chapter 12

Fig. 2.4 Confusion.

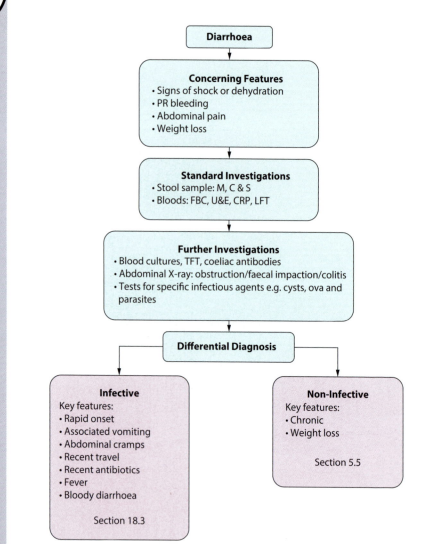

Fig. 2.5 Diarrhoea.

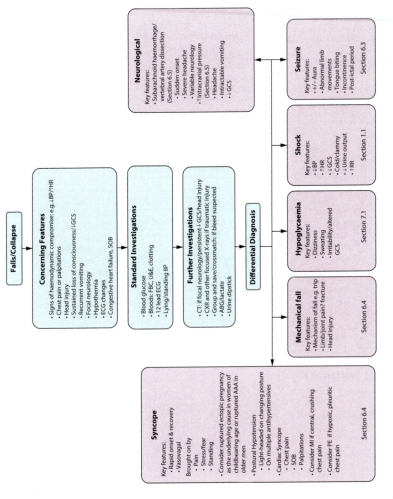

Falls/Collapse

Concerning Features
- Signs of haemodynamic compromise: e.g. ↓BP/↑HR
- Chest pain or palpitations
- Head injury
- Sustained loss of consciousness/↓GCS
- Recurrent vomiting
- Focal neurology
- Hypothermia
- ECG changes
- Congestive heart failure, SOB

Standard Investigations
- Blood glucose
- Bloods: FBC, U&E, clotting
- 12 lead ECG
- Lying/standing BP

Further Investigations
- CT: if focal neurology/persistent ↓GCS/head injury
- CXR and other focused X-rays if traumatic injury
- Group and save/crossmatch: if bleed suspected
- ABG/lactate
- Urine dipstick

Differential Diagnosis

Syncope
Key features:
- Rapid onset & recovery
- Vasovagal
Brought on by
- Pain
- Stress/fear
- Standing
- Consider ruptured ectopic pregnancy as the underlying cause in women of childbearing age or ruptured AAA in older men
- Postural Hypotension
- Light-headed on changing posture
- On multiple antihypertensives
- Cardiac Syncope
- Chest pain
- SOB
- Palpitations
- Consider MI if central, crushing chest pain
- Consider PE if hypoxic, pleuritic chest pain

Section 6.4

Mechanical fall
Key features:
- Mechanism of fall e.g. trip
- Limb/joint pain? fracture
- Head injury

Section 6.4

Hypoglycaemia
Key features:
- Dizziness
- Sweating
- Irritability/altered GCS

Section 7.1

Shock
Key features:
- ↓BP
- ↑HR
- ↓GCS
- Cold/clammy
- ↓Urine output
- ↑RR

Section 1.1

Seizure
Key features:
- +/– Aura
- Abnormal limb movements
- Tongue biting
- Incontinence
- Post-ictal period

Section 6.3

Neurological
Key features:
- Subarachnoid haemorrhage/vertebral artery dissection (Section 6.5)
- Sudden onset
- Severe headache
- Variable neurology
- ↑Intracranial pressure (Section 6.5)
- Headache
- Intractable vomiting
- ↓GCS

Fig. 2.6 Falls/collapse.

Emergency and acute medicine

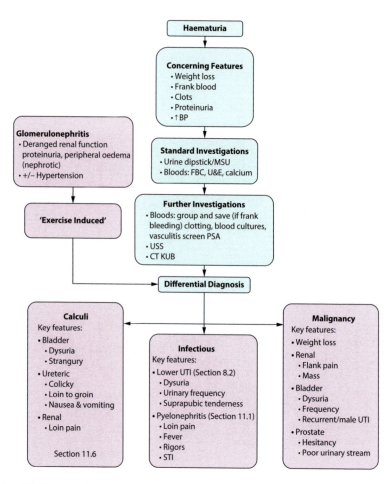

Fig. 2.7 Haematuria.

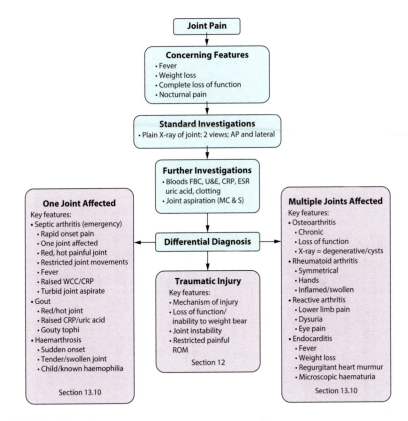

Fig. 2.8 Joint pain.

Emergency and acute medicine

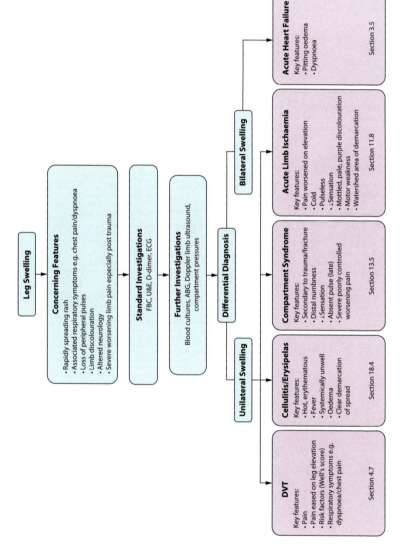

Leg Swelling

Concerning Features
• Rapidly spreading rash
• Associated respiratory symptoms e.g. chest pain/dyspnoea
• Loss of peripheral pulses
• Limb discolouration
• Altered neurology
• Severe worsening limb pain especially post trauma

Standard Investigations
FBC, U&E, D-dimer, ECG

Further Investigations
Blood cultures, ABG, Doppler limb ultrasound, compartment pressures

Differential Diagnosis

Unilateral Swelling

Bilateral Swelling

DVT
Key features:
• Pain
• Pain eased on leg elevation
• Risk factors (Well's score)
• Respiratory symptoms e.g. dyspnoea/chest pain

Section 4.7

Cellulitis/Erysipelas
Key features:
• Hot, erythematous
• Fever
• Systemically unwell
• Oedema
• Clear demarcation of spread

Section 18.4

Compartment Syndrome
Key features:
• Secondary to trauma/fracture
• Distal numbness
• ↓Sensation
• Absent pulse (late)
• Severe poorly controlled worsening pain

Section 13.5

Acute Limb Ischaemia
Key features:
• Pain worsened on elevation
• Cold
• Pulseless
• ↓Sensation
• Mottled, pale, purple discolouration
• Motor weakness
• Watershed area of demarcation

Section 11.8

Acute Heart Failure
Key features:
• Pitting oedema
• Dyspnoea

Section 3.5

Fig. 2.9 Leg swelling.

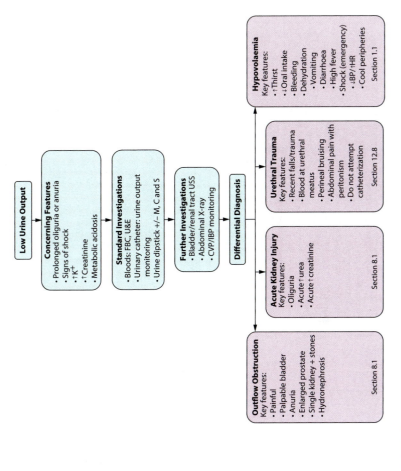

Low Urine Output

Concerning Features
- Prolonged oliguria or anuria
- Signs of shock
- ↑K⁺
- ↑Creatinine
- Metabolic acidosis

Standard Investigations
- Bloods: FBC, U&E
- Urinary catheter: urine output monitoring
- Urine dipstick +/- M, C and S

Further Investigations
- Bladder/renal tract USS
- Abdominal X-ray
- CVP/IBP monitoring

Differential Diagnosis

Outflow Obstruction
Key features:
- Painful
- Palpable bladder
- Anuria
- Enlarged prostate
- Single kidney + stones
- Hydronephrosis

Section 8.1

Acute Kidney Injury
Key features:
- Oliguria
- Acute ↑ urea
- Acute ↑ creatinine

Section 8.1

Urethral Trauma
Key features:
- Recent falls/trauma
- Blood at urethral meatus
- Perineal bruising
- Abdominal pain with peritonism
- Do not attempt catheterization

Section 12.8

Hypovolaemia
Key features:
- ↑Thirst
- ↓Oral intake
- Bleeding
- Dehydration
- Vomiting
- Diarrhoea
- High fever
- Shock (emergency)
- ↓BP/↑HR
- Cool peripheries

Section 1.1

Fig. 2.10 Low urine output.

Emergency and acute medicine

Emergency and acute medicine

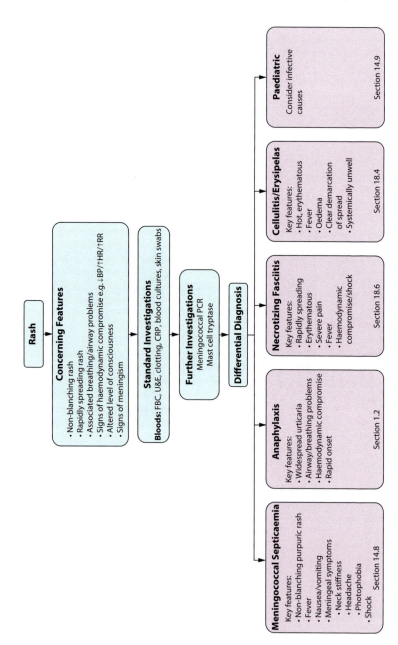

Rash

Concerning Features
· Non-blanching rash
· Rapidly spreading rash
· Associated breathing/airway problems
· Signs of haemodynamic compromise e.g. ↓BP/↑HR/↑RR
· Altered level of consciousness
· Signs of meningism

Standard Investigations
Bloods: FBC, U&E, clotting, CRP, blood cultures, skin swabs

Further Investigations
Meningococcal PCR
Mast cell tryptase

Differential Diagnosis

Meningococcal Septicaemia
Key features:
· Non-blanching purpuric rash
· Fever
· Nausea/vomiting
· Meningeal symptoms
  · Neck stiffness
  · Headache
  · Photophobia
· Shock   Section 14.8

Anaphylaxis
Key features:
· Widespread urticaria
· Airway/breathing problems
· Haemodynamic compromise
· Rapid onset

            Section 1.2

Necrotizing Fasciitis
Key features:
· Rapidly spreading
· Erythematous
· Severe pain
· Fever
· Haemodynamic compromise/shock

            Section 18.6

Cellulitis/Erysipelas
Key features:
· Hot, erythematous
· Fever
· Oedema
· Clear demarcation of spread
· Systemically unwell

            Section 18.4

Paediatric
Consider infective causes

            Section 14.9

Fig. 2.11 Rash.

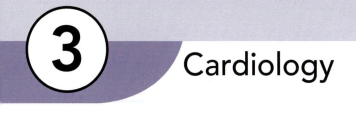

3 Cardiology

3.1 CHEST PAIN

Aetiology

- Cardiac:
    - Acute coronary syndrome (ACS)
    - ST elevation myocardial infarction (STEMI)
    - Non-ST elevation myocardial infarction (NSTEMI)
    - Unstable angina
    - Aortic dissection
    - Stable angina
    - Arrhythmias
    - Pericarditis/myocarditis
- Respiratory:
    - Pulmonary embolism (PE)
    - Pneumothorax and tension pneumothorax
    - Pneumonia
    - Bronchial carcinoma
    - Pleural effusion/empyema
- Gastrointestinal:
    - Gastro-oesophageal reflux
    - Oesophageal reflux/spasm or rupture
    - Hiatus hernia
    - Biliary tract disease
    - Pancreatitis
    - Perforated peptic ulcer
- Musculoskeletal:
    - Costochondritis
    - Fibromyalgia
    - Minor trauma/rib fracture
    - Shingles
    - Bony metastases

- Psychological:
  - Anxiety
  - Depression

Clinical features

- Table 3.1

Table 3.1 **Causes of chest pain**

DIFFERENTIAL DIAGNOSIS	FEATURES OF PAIN

Acute coronary syndromes (ACSs)
  STEMI
  NSTEMI
  Unstable angina
	• Heavy, crushing pressure
	• Central
	• Radiates to jaw, either arm or shoulders

Stable angina	• Similar character to ACS • Exertional • Always relieved by rest ± GTN
Pericarditis	• Sharp • Anterior • Well-localized • Exacerbated by lying down • Alleviated by sitting forward
Pulmonary embolism	• Pleuritic (inspiratory) • Sharp

ACUTE CORONARY SYNDROMES

Definition

- A spectrum of clinical presentations of unstable coronary artery disease encompassing partial to complete rupture and thrombosis of an atheromatous plaque in an artery
- STEMI: Cardiac-sounding chest pain associated with ST elevation on an ECG in an anatomically contiguous pattern
- NSTEMI: Cardiac-sounding chest pain lasting 15 min or more which may or may not be associated with ischaemic ECG changes, but causes an elevation in troponin
- Unstable angina (UA): Cardiac-sounding chest pain for 15 min or more, which may be associated with dynamic ECG changes with no troponin rise

---

MICRO-reference

NICE Guidelines for NSTEMI and Unstable Angina, http://www.nice.org.uk/nicemedia/live/12949/47924/47924.pdf

> **MICRO-print**
> **Other causes of a raised troponin**
> - Sepsis
> - Aortic dissection
> - PE
> - Myocarditis/pericarditis
> - Cardiac failure
> - Renal failure
> - Stroke

Clinical features

- Pain in chest and/or pain in arms (particularly left), back or jaw >15 min
- Chest tightness/heaviness
- Autonomic symptoms, e.g. nausea, vomiting, sweating
- Breathlessness
- History of ischaemic heart disease or risk factors for the condition
- Haemodynamic instability
- Not relieved with rest or GTN

Investigations

- 12-lead ECG (see Fig. 3.1)

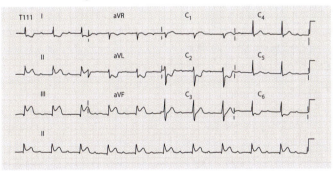

Fig. 3.1 ECG of STEMI.

- Blood tests:
    - FBC: may show neutrophilia, anaemia can exacerbate stable angina
    - U&E: assess for renal impairment
    - LFT: may be deranged if right heart failure
    - Coagulation screen if considering commencing anticoagulation
- Cardiac markers:
    - Troponin I or T is gold standard
    - High-sensitivity troponins (HSTn) allow for more accurate detection (see Table 3.2)

Table 3.2 **Comparison of STEMI and NSTEMI, unstable angina**

CONDITION	PAIN CHARACTER	ECG FINDINGS	TROPONIN RESULT
STEMI	Ischaemic	• Hyperacute T waves may be seen in early MI • ST elevation • New left bundle branch block (LBBB)	Raised troponin I or T at 12 h or earlier if high-sensitivity troponin
NSTEMI	Ischaemic	• ST depression • T wave inversion • ECG may be normal	Raised troponin I or T at 12 h or earlier if high-sensitivity troponin
Unstable angina	Ischaemic	• ST depression • T wave inversion • ECG may be normal	Normal troponin at 12 h or earlier if high-sensitivity troponin

- A 6 h cutoff threshold may be used for some HSTn assays to exclude STEMI/NSTEMI if negative
- CK-MB used in some centres, but less specific than troponins
- CXR: look for evidence of pulmonary oedema complicating MI and to exclude other causes of pain
- Consider echocardiogram: assess for areas of hypokinesis, biventricular function and valve abnormalities
- Further tests:
  - Angiogram: gold standard for assessing coronary artery disease and chamber pressures
  - Exercise treadmill test/stress echo/myoview: assess for reversible ischaemia
  - CT/MR angiogram less invasive but less sensitive test to view coronary arteries

---

MICRO-facts

High-sensitivity troponin T or I (HSTn)
- New, sensitive assays to detect even very small troponin rise
- Most assays detect a rise in troponin within 6 h of symptoms; therefore if negative at this time, NSTEMI can be excluded – consult local guidelines
- Low-level elevation common in elderly/patients with comorbidities
  - If elevated, repeat test in a further 6 h
  - Further increase of e.g. >50% (consult local guidelines as assays differ) would then indicate NSTEMI

Management

● See Fig. 3.2

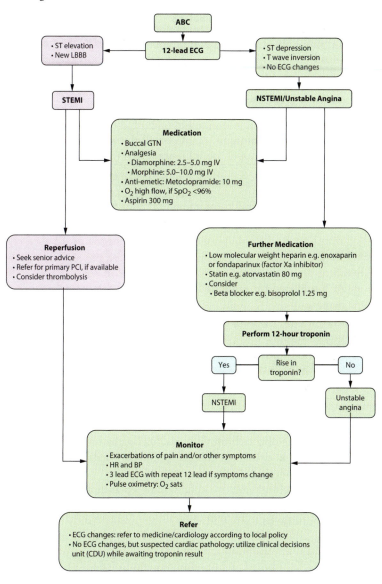

Fig. 3.2 Management of acute coronary syndromes.

Contraindications to thrombolysis

- See Table 3.3

Table 3.3 **Contraindications to thrombolysis**

ABSOLUTE	RELATIVE
Patient refusal	Ischaemic stroke/TIA >12 months
History of haemorrhagic stroke	Recent head injury
Major trauma/surgery <2 weeks	Chronic warfarin therapy
Aortic dissection	Chronic renal/liver disease
Uncontrolled high blood pressure (>180/100 mmHg)	Controlled severe HTN (systolic 180 mmHg)
Bleeding diathesis (tendency)	Active peptic ulcer
Active bleeding <10/7	History of GI haemorrhage
Known bleeding disorder	Pregnancy

Secondary prevention

- ABACS:
    - ACE inhibitor, e.g. ramipril 1.25 mg OD (to be uptitrated as an outpatient)
    - Beta-blocker, e.g. bisoprolol 1.25 mg OD (to be uptitrated as an outpatient)
    - Aspirin 75 mg OD
    - Clopidogrel 75 mg OD for 1 year if NSTEMI
    - Statin, e.g. atorvastatin 80 mg ON

Complications of MI

- Further chest pain/rest pain
- Arrhythmias: including tachyarrhythmias, bradyarrhythmias, heart block
- Cardiogenic shock: circulatory collapse, pulmonary oedema, hypotension
- Left ventricular aneurysm
- Mechanical complications: ventricular wall or septal rupture, papillary muscle rupture resulting in acute mitral regurgitation
- Congestive cardiac failure (CCF)

PERICARDITIS

Definitions

- Pericarditis: inflammation of the pericardium
- Myocarditis: inflammation of the myocardium (commonly occurs concurrently with pericarditis)
- Myopericarditis: symptoms of pericarditis and ECG changes ± troponin rise

Aetiology
- Idiopathic
- Secondary to infection:
  - Viral:
    - Influenzae
    - Coxsackie
    - Parvovirus
    - Epstein-Barr
    - HIV
  - Bacterial:
    - *Streptococcus pneumoniae*
    - Rheumatic fever
    - TB
    - *Staphylococcus aureus*
  - Fungal

> **MICRO-facts**
>
> Pericarditis commonly presents following a viral illness.

- Post-MI: acute or after a few weeks (Dressler's syndrome)
- Iatrogenic:
  - Penicillins
  - Procainamide
- Secondary to chronic illness:
  - Rheumatoid arthritis
  - Systemic lupus erythematous (SLE)
  - Malignancy
  - Sarcoidosis

Clinical features
- Pleuritic chest pain
- Sharp in character and usually well localized
- ↑ Pain on lying down
- ↓ Pain sitting forward

Investigations
- ECG:
  - Saddle-shaped ST elevation
  - Pattern of ST elevation does not fit with a particular coronary artery territory
  - No reciprocal ST depression

Emergency and acute medicine

- Bloods:
  - ↑ WCC
  - ↑ ESR/CRP
  - Troponin may be elevated if concurrent myocarditis
- Echo: may show e.g. pericardial effusion

> **MICRO-print**
> - The pericardium contains no contractile cells; therefore pericarditis with no myocardial involvement does not have ECG changes.
> - Myocarditis may have ECG changes and raised troponin.

Management

- Pain relief: NSAIDs, paracetamol, weak opiates
- Reassurance: pericarditis usually settles within 4 weeks but recurrence is common

AORTIC DISSECTION

Definition

- Tear within the layers of the aortic wall causing blood to flow within the intima-media space, causing separation

Clinical features

- Pain: abrupt, tearing/ripping, interscapular
- Syncope
- Weak peripheral pulses
- Hypertension or history of hypertension
- Patient may be hypotensive due to blood loss
- Features of stroke if brachiocephalic or left common carotid involvement
- If proximal aorta affected, the following may occur:
  - Aortic regurgitation
  - Cardiac tamponade
  - MI

Investigation

- ECG: features of left ventricular hypertrophy, ischaemia, or may be normal
- CXR:
  - Widened mediastinum
  - 'Double knuckle' aorta
  - Deviated trachea
  - Calcified aorta
  - Unilateral pleural effusion
- Blood tests: FBC, U&E, glucose, coagulation, cross-match 6–8 units
- Imaging to confirm diagnosis, e.g. CT, MRA, echocardiogram

Management

- See Fig. 3.3

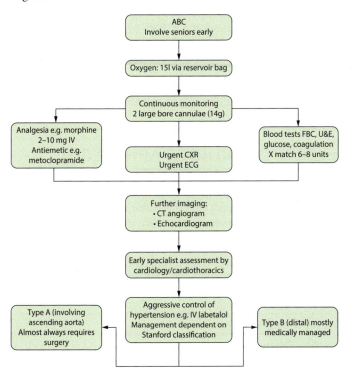

Fig. 3.3 Management of aortic dissection.

MICRO-case

A 54-year-old man is brought to the ED by ambulance after he experienced severe central chest pain at work. The ambulance was called and arrived within 10 min, at which time he was still in pain. He is responsive, breathing and has a BP of 130/70 mmHg. He has two IV cannulae in situ and high-flow oxygen is applied via a mask. In the ambulance he also received sublingual nitrate.

In the ED he was given 300 mg aspirin, 300 mg clopidogrel and 5 mg morphine along with metoclopramide. He is now more comfortable but continues to look pale. His oxygen saturations are 98% on high-flow oxygen with a respiratory rate of 18 breaths per minute. An ECG is recorded showing some ischaemic changes but no ST elevation.

continued...

continued...

> **Key points:**
> - This patient is most likely to be having a NSTEMI.
> - This patient could develop a STEMI, which may require PCI; therefore it is important to do continuous ECG monitoring.
> - Continuous ECG monitoring is also important to identify life-threatening arrhythmias early.
> - Treat with fondaparinux/low molecular weight heparin (LMWH).
> - In a patient with this presentation, troponin should be checked according to local protocol.

3.2 ELECTROCARDIOGRAPHY (ECG)

Definition

- A standard ECG has 12 leads which produce individual tracings comparing the spread of electrical depolarization across the heart
- See Table 3.4

Table 3.4 **Area of the heart and its corresponding chest lead**

AREA OF THE HEART	LEAD
Right atrium	aVR
Anterior surface (right ventricle/septum)	V1–4
Lateral surface (left ventricle)	V5–6, aVL, I
Inferior surface	II, III, aVF

- ECG interpretation (See Fig. 3.4 and Table 3.5)

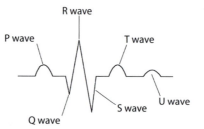

Fig. 3.4 Normal ECG.

Table 3.5 **ECG interpretation with normal values**

ECG	NORMAL VALUES
Rate	60–100 bpm Large square 0.2 s Small square 0.04 s
Rhythm	Sinus: P wave before every QRS complex

Cardiac axis	Normal axis:
	  −30 to +90
	  I and aVF + ve
	  I and II + ve and aVF − ve

P waves	P wave before QRS complex
PR interval	0.12–0.2 s (3–5 small squares)
QRS complex	<0.12 s (<3 small squares)
ST segment	Level with baseline
T waves	Upright in V3 to V6

MICRO-facts

Serial ECGs are invaluable to guide patient management.

3.3 PALPITATIONS

Definition

- Sensation/awareness of one's own heartbeat

Causes

- Sinus tachycardia
- Ectopic beats
- Atrial fibrillation
- Atrial flutter
- Atrio-ventricular re-entrant tachycardia (AVRT)
- Atrio-ventricular nodal re-entrant tachycardia (AVRNT)
- Ventricular tachycardia

Clinical features

- Asymptomatic
- Dizziness
- Presyncope/syncope
- Dyspnoea
- Chest pain

Investigations

- All patients with palpitations ± other symptoms
- ECG: ideally during episode or 24 h recording
- Blood tests:
    - FBC: anaemia
    - U&Es, calcium and magnesium: electrolyte derangement can precipitate arrhythmias
    - Thyroid function tests (TFTs): hyperthyroidism can lead to tachycardia and AF
- Other investigations are dependent on careful clinical history and examination

SINUS TACHYCARDIA

Definition

- Fast heart rate >100 bpm
- Sinus rhythm: normal P wave morphology
- QRS complexes: regular and narrow

Causes

- Exercise
- Pain
- Anxiety
- Anaemia
- Fever
- Sepsis
- Hypoxia
- Hypovolaemia
- Stimulants: nicotine, caffeine
- Drugs: atropine, salbutamol
- Recreational drugs: cocaine, amphetamines, ecstasy, GHB
- Pulmonary embolus (PE)

ATRIAL FIBRILLATION

Classification of AF

- See Table 3.6

Table 3.6 **Classification of AF**

CLASSIFICATION	CHARACTERISTICS
Paroxysmal	Episodes • Last <7 days but usually <24 h • Recur again after an interval • Terminate spontaneously

(Continued)

Table 3.6 *(Continued)* **Classification of AF**

CLASSIFICATION	CHARACTERISTICS
Persistent	Episodes • Last >7 days • Recur again after an interval
Permanent	Continuous AF Failed/unattempted cardioversion

Causes

- Hypertension
- Ischaemic heart disease/myocardial infarction
- Thyrotoxicosis
- Valvular heart disease
- Alcohol
- Sepsis
- Pulmonary embolism
- Post-cardiac surgery
- Pericarditis/myocarditis

Clinical features

- Palpitations
- Dyspnoea
- Chest pain
- Dizziness/syncope
- Irregularly irregular pulse
- Hypotension
- Precipitant disease, e.g. hyperthyroidism, PE
- Embolic sequelae, e.g. stroke, TIA

Investigations

- See Table 3.7

Table 3.7 **Investigations of AF**

INVESTIGATION	FINDINGS
ECG	• Absent P waves (see Fig. 3.5) • Irregularly irregular QRS rate
Blood tests	• Raised WCC (if precipitated by infection) • Deranged TFTs (if precipitated by hyperthyroidism) • Deranged electrolytes – hypokalaemia and hypomagnesaemia in particular may precipitate AF

(Continued)

Emergency and acute medicine

Table 3.7 *(Continued)* **Investigations of AF**

INVESTIGATION	FINDINGS
Chest X-ray	• Heart size – atrial enlargement predisposes to AF • Pulmonary oedema • Underlying precipitant disease, e.g. pneumonia
Echocardiogram	• Left ventricular impairment • Atrial enlargement • Valve lesion, e.g. mitral stenosis may predispose to AF

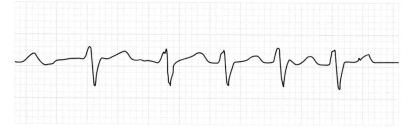

Fig. 3.5 ECG of atrial fibrillation.

Management

- See Fig. 3.6.
- If unstable, proceed to emergency-synchronized DC shock after sedation – seek senior help.
- If stable, consider rate vs. rhythm control strategy with senior input.
  - Note there is no prognostic benefit to being in sinus rhythm rather than AF.
  - Any patient who has had AF should be risk stratified with e.g. CHADS2 score (see MICRO-facts) and offered appropriate anticoagulation.
    - The risk of stroke persists even if patient is returned to sinus rhythm.

MICRO-facts

CHADS2-VASc score: evaluates ischaemic stroke risk in patients with AF without warfarin treatment

Congestive heart failure	1
Hypertension	1
Age >75 years	2

continued...

continued...

Diabetes Mellitus	1
Previous Stroke, TIA or TE	2
Vascular disease (prior MI, peripheral arterial disease or aortic plaque)	1
Aged 65–74 years	1
Sex category (female)	1
Maximum score:	9

Score:

0	–	low risk
1	–	moderate risk
>2	–	high risk

Lane DA, Lip GY. Use of the CHADS2-VASc and HAS-BLED scores to aid decision making for thromboprophylaxis in non valvular atrial fibrillation. *Circulation.* 2012 August 14; 126 (7): 860–5.

- To pursue a rhythm control strategy, the onset of patient symptoms must be <48 h.
  - Uncertain duration or >48 h means the patient is at risk of embolic stroke if electrically or chemically cardioverted.
  - In this case, discuss with cardiology.
    - May have transoesophageal echocardiography to rule out left atrial thrombus followed by cardioversion if urgent management required.
    - Otherwise, may be anticoagulated for 4–6 weeks and then cardioverted.

MICRO-facts

Electrical cardioversion is the treatment for unstable AF.

MICRO-reference
NICE Guidelines: CG36 Atrial Fibrillation: Full Guideline, http://guidance.nice.org.uk/CG36/Guidance/pdf/English

Resuscitation Council UK: Adult Tachycardia (with Pulse) Algorithm, https://www.resus.org.uk/pages/periarst.pdf

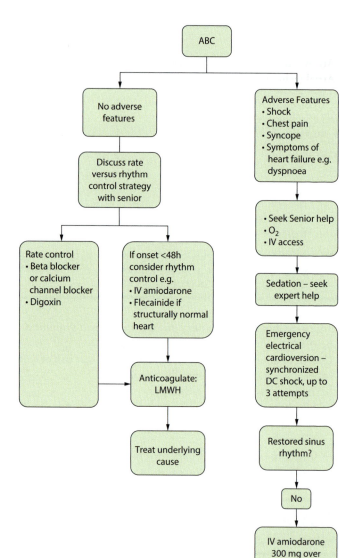

Fig. 3.6 Management of AF.

REGULAR NARROW-COMPLEX TACHYCARDIAS

Definition

- Rate: >100 bpm
- Narrow QRS complex: <120 ms

- Include:
    - Atrioventricular node re-entrant tachycardia (AVNRT)
    - Atrioventricular reciprocating tachycardia (AVRT)
    - Atrial tachycardias
    - Atrial flutter
    - Exclude sinus tachycardia with careful ECG interpretation

Investigations

- ECG
- Bloods: FBC, U&Es (K+, Ca, Mg imbalance can induce AVNRT), TFTs (hyperthyroidism can induce AVNRT), digoxin levels (if appropriate)
- CXR

Management

- See Fig. 3.7

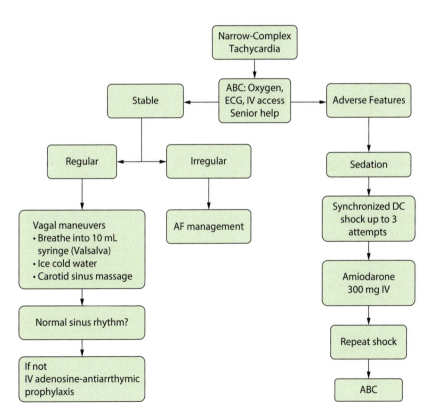

Fig. 3.7 Management of narrow-complex tachycardia.

> **MICRO-reference**
> Adapted from the Resuscitation Council Guidelines (UK), www.resus.org.uk/

Long-term management

- For atrial flutter, elective synchronized DC cardioversion has a good success rate for terminating the arrhythmia.
- Radiofrequency ablation
  - For recurrent attacks of AVRT/AVNRT/atrial flutter.
  - High-frequency alternating current is used to ablate the dysfunctional conducting tissue, under image guidance.
- Precipitating factors: reduce alcohol and caffeine intake.
- Optimize management of comorbidities: cardiovascular disease.
- Rate-limiting therapy such as beta-blockade may be used as prophylaxis for these arrhythmias.
- Anticoagulation is not required for AVNRT or AVRT, unlike for AF.

VENTRICULAR TACHYCARDIA

Definition

- Rate: >100 bpm, usually in excess of 150 bpm
- Broad QRS complex: >120 ms
- AV dissociation

Causes

- IHD
- Structural heart disease
- MI
- Electrolyte disturbance: hypokalaemia, hypomagnesemia, hypocalcaemia

Clinical features

- VT with a pulse:
  - Patient often acutely unwell
  - Chest pain
  - Dyspnoea
  - Diaphoresis
  - Palpitations
  - Nausea
  - Syncope/presyncope
  - May be asymptomatic
- Pulseless VT: medical emergency (follow arrest guidelines, Fig. 1.2)

Investigations

- 12-lead ECG (See Fig. 3.8)

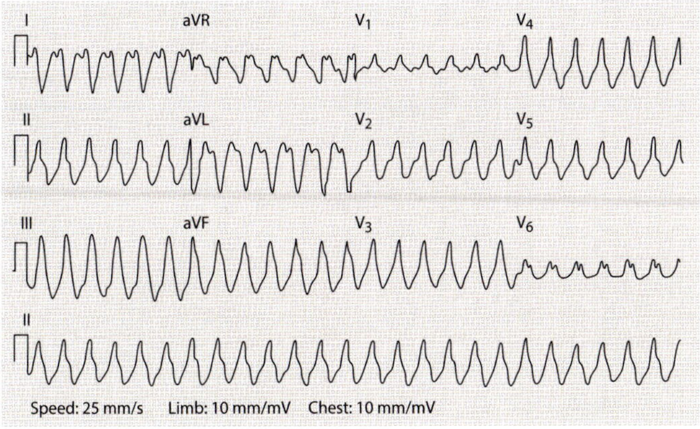

Fig. 3.8 ECG of VT.

- Continuous cardiac and vital sign monitoring
- Bloods: FBC, U&Es, LFTs, serum Mg^{2+}, TFTs, cardiac enzymes

---

MICRO-facts

Broad complex tachycardias

- Patients with pre-existing bundle branch block who have a tachycardia may be mistaken for having VT.
- If they have co-existent AF the two conditions may be particularly difficult to distinguish.
- Seek expert advice in these situations, but assume VT until proven otherwise.

Management

- See Fig. 3.9
- Cardioversion to restore sinus rhythm as soon as possible:
  - Pharmacological, e.g. amiodarone
  - Electrical: DC shock

Further management

- After restoring sinus rhythm
- Continuous monitoring
- Repeat ECG
- Bloods:
  - Monitor electrolytes
  - Troponin; although elevation does not always indicate MI as a cause
- Treat reversible cause
- Echocardiogram

Emergency and acute medicine

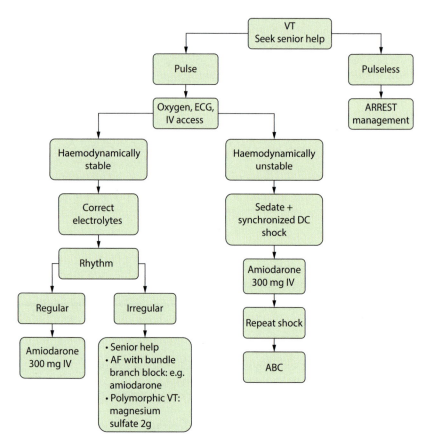

Fig 3.9 Management of VT.

- Long-term anti-arrhythmic therapy, e.g. beta-blockers or amiodarone
- Implanted cardiac defibrillator (ICD)

> **MICRO-reference**
> Adapted from the Resuscitation Council Guidelines (UK), www.resus.org.uk/

3.4 BRADYCARDIA

Definition

- Slow heart rate <60 bpm

Emergency and acute medicine

Causes

- Sinus bradycardia:
  - Physical fitness
  - Hypothyroidism
  - Hypothermia
  - Hypoglycaemia
  - Drugs: beta-blockers, calcium-channel blockers
- First-degree heart block
- Sick sinus syndrome
- Second degree heart block
- Complete (third degree) heart block

Investigations

- See Fig. 3.10

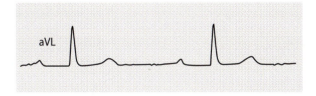

Fig. 3.10 ECG of first degree HB.

Clinical features

- Palpitations
- Blackouts
- Dizziness
- Chest pain
- Exercise intolerance
- Breathlessness

Investigations

- See Fig. 3.10

Management

- See Fig. 3.11

MICRO-reference
Adapted from the Resuscitation Council Guidelines (UK), www.resus.org.uk/

Emergency and acute medicine

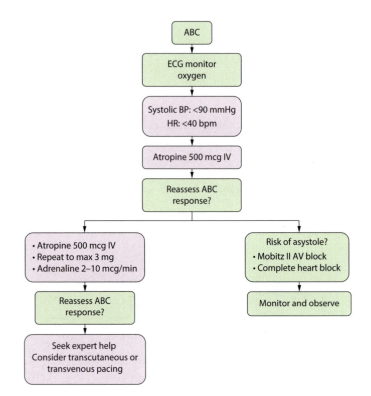

Fig. 3.11 Management of bradycardia.

3.5 ACUTE HEART FAILURE

Aetiology

● See Table 3.8

Table 3.8 **Causes of heart failure: comparison of low and high cardiac outputs**

LOW CARDIAC OUTPUT	HIGH CARDIAC OUTPUT
Pump failure	Hyperthyroidism
Left ventricular dysfunction	Paget's disease
Ischaemic heart disease (IHD)	Chronic anaemia
Myocardial infarction (MI)	Pregnancy
Cardiomyopathy	
Poor outflow	
Valve disease	
Hypertension	
Arrhythmia	

Clinical features

- Acute SOB
- Orthopnoea
- Paroxysmal nocturnal dyspnoea
- Sputum: pink, frothy
- Pallor and sweating
- ↑ HR
- ↑ RR
- ↑ JVP
- Lung crackles: pulmonary oedema
- Oedema: peripheral, sacral
- Wheeze: cardiac asthma

Investigations

- ECG: arrhythmias, ischaemic changes, LBBB, RBBB
- CXR: ABCDE (see Fig. 3.12 and MICRO-fact box)
- ABG
- Echocardiogram
- Bloods:
  - FBC: anaemia
  - U&Es: check renal function
  - Troponin: although elevation does not always indicate MI as a cause
  - Albumin: hypoalbuminaemia in pulmonary oedema
  - BNP: used in some centres to aid diagnosis of heart failure

---

MICRO-facts

Features to look for on a CXR of acute heart failure:
- Alveolar bat wings
- Kerley B lines
- Cardiomegaly
- Diversion of veins in upper lobes
- Effusions

Management

- ABC
- Keep patient upright
- Oxygen
- IV access
- Drug treatment:
  - Diamorphine 2.5–5 mg IV: pain relief, vasodilator
  - Furosemide 40–80 mg IV to relieve pulmonary oedema
  - Nitrate sublingual and/or IV: vasodilatory

Emergency and acute medicine

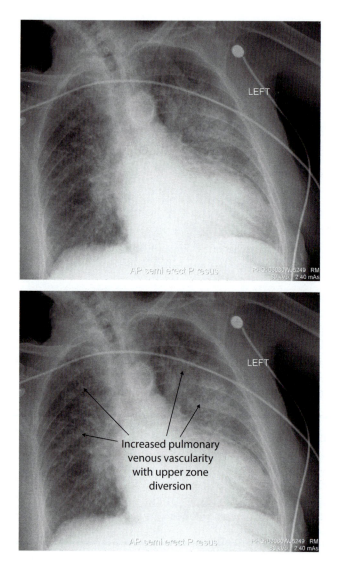

Fig. 3.12 Chest X-ray of acute heart failure.

- Non-invasive positive pressure ventilation (NIPPV): CPAP
- Daily U&E and weight; strict fluid balance
- If BP drops = cardiogenic shock
- ABC

- Inotropes: ↑ cardiac contractility
  - Dobutamine
  - Adrenaline
  - Noradrenaline

Long-term management

- Improve prognosis:
  - ACE inhibitors
  - Beta-blockers: caution in acute management
  - Spironolactone/eplerenone
- Improve symptoms:
  - Diuretics

MICRO-reference

NICE Guidelines for Chronic Heart Failure, http://www.nice.org.uk/nicemedia/live/13099/50526/50526.pdf

---

MICRO-case

An 89-year-old man is brought to the ED after waking up in the night gasping for breath. On arrival, he is sweating, very pale and very short of breath. He is given high-flow oxygen via a mask and sat upright. IV access is obtained and an ECG monitor is connected. His other observations are as follows: BP, 110/80; HR, 105; RR, 21; oxygen saturations of 91% on 15 L oxygen. On examination, crackles can be heard bilaterally in the bases of his chest and he has a displaced apex beat to the sixth intercostal space in the mid-axillary line. He also has pitting oedema in both of his ankles. The patient is given 80 mg furosemide and is put on an IV infusion of GTN. A CXR is requested that shows bilateral shadowing, cardiomegaly and effusions at the costophrenic angles.

- This patient is suffering from acute-on-chronic heart failure.
- The chronic heart failure is indicated by the swollen ankles and displaced apex beat.
- It is important to keep the patient sat upright to aid breathing.
- A systolic BP <100 may indicate cardiogenic shock.
- Examination should be performed to look for a cause. Do not let this delay treatment for the patient.
- Give high-dose furosemide and monitor its effect, i.e. oxygen sats, respiratory rate, listen to chest. If the patient is not improving, then give another dose of furosemide or consider a continuous IV infusion.
- Consider NIV (CPAP) if patient continues to be dyspnoeic despite treatment.

3.6 SEVERE HYPERTENSION

Definition
- Systolic BP >200 bpm, diastolic BP >120 bpm

Aetiology
- Uncontrolled essential hypertension
- Phaeochromocytoma
- Thyrotoxic storm
- Cushing's reflex ($\uparrow$ intracranial pressure)
- Pre-eclampsia/eclampsia

Clinical features
- Chest pain
- Arrhythmias
- Headache
- Epistaxis
- Light-headedness
- Anxiety
- Altered mental state (hypertensive encephalopathy)
- Vomiting

Signs of end-organ damage
- See Table 3.9

Table 3.9 **Signs of end-organ damage**

END-ORGAN DAMAGE	FEATURES

Retinal	• Opthalmoscopy:
	  • Exudates
	  • Haemorrhages
	  • Papilloedema

Renal	• Blood tests: deranged U&E
	• Urinalysis:
	  • Blood
	  • Protein

Cardiac	• ECG: left ventricular hypertrophy

Management
- See Fig. 3.13

Indications for admission
- Diastolic BP persistently >125 mmHg
- Retinal haemorrhages

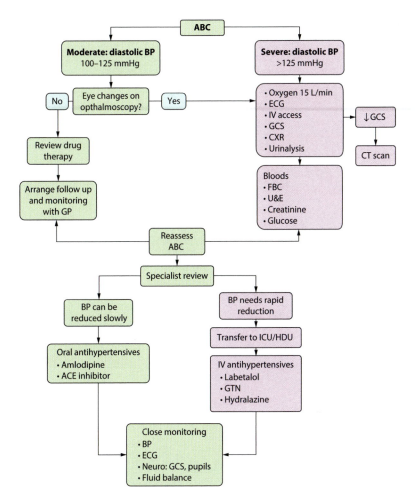

Fig. 3.13 Management of severe hypertension.

- New/worsening renal impairment
- Confusion

Indications to rapidly reduce BP

- Eclampsia
- MI
- Aortic dissection
- Hypertensive encephalopathy

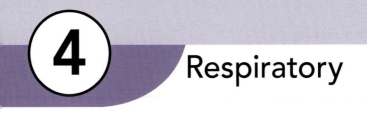

4 Respiratory

4.1 ARTERIAL BLOOD GASES (ABGs)

Definition

- Analysis of arterial blood to assess:
  - Blood pH
  - Partial pressure of oxygen (PaO_2)
  - Partial pressure of carbon dioxide ($PaCO_2$)
  - Serum bicarbonate $\left(HCO_3^-\right)$
  - Many machines also have carboxyhaemaglobin, estimated haemoglobin, electrolytes and anion gap

---

> **MICRO-facts**
>
> **Normal values:**
>
> | | |
> |---|---|
> | pH | 7.35–7.45 |
> | PaO_2 | 11–13 kPa |
> | $PaCO_2$ | 4.7–6.0 kPa |
> | HCO_3^- | 22–28 mmol/L |
> | Base excess | –2 to +2 mmol/L |
> | Anion gap | 12–16 mmol/L |

Respiratory indications

- Dyspnoea
- Low SpO_2
- Tachypnoea
- Suspected respiratory illness

Contraindications

- Poor collateral circulation – perform Allen test to check
- Previous vessel harvesting, e.g. coronary artery bypass grafting (CABG)
- Arteriovenous fistula

Interpretation

- Follow the steps in Fig. 4.1

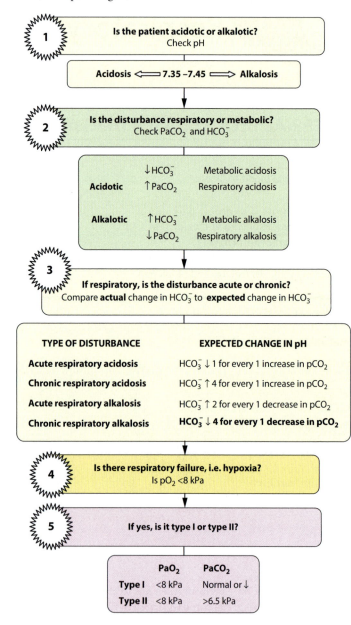

1 Is the patient acidotic or alkalotic?
Check pH

Acidosis ⟸ 7.35–7.45 ⟹ Alkalosis

2 Is the disturbance respiratory or metabolic?
Check $PaCO_2$ and HCO_3^-

	$\downarrow HCO_3^-$	Metabolic acidosis
Acidotic	$\uparrow PaCO_2$	Respiratory acidosis
Alkalotic	$\uparrow HCO_3^-$	Metabolic alkalosis
	$\downarrow PaCO_2$	Respiratory alkalosis

3 If respiratory, is the disturbance acute or chronic?
Compare **actual** change in HCO_3^- to **expected** change in HCO_3^-

TYPE OF DISTURBANCE	EXPECTED CHANGE IN pH
Acute respiratory acidosis	$HCO_3^- \downarrow 1$ for every 1 increase in pCO_2
Chronic respiratory acidosis	$HCO_3^- \uparrow 4$ for every 1 increase in pCO_2
Acute respiratory alkalosis	$HCO_3^- \uparrow 2$ for every 1 decrease in pCO_2
Chronic respiratory alkalosis	$HCO_3^- \downarrow 4$ for every 1 decrease in pCO_2

4 Is there respiratory failure, i.e. hypoxia?
Is $pO_2 < 8$ kPa

5 If yes, is it type I or type II?

	PaO_2	$PaCO_2$
Type I	<8 kPa	Normal or $\downarrow$
Type II	<8 kPa	>6.5 kPa

Fig. 4.1 ABG interpretation in a patient with suspected respiratory disease.

Emergency and acute medicine

RESPIRATORY FAILURE

- Common causes of type I vs. type II respiratory failure are shown in Table 4.1

Table 4.1 **Common causes of type I vs. type II respiratory failure**

TYPE I	TYPE II
Asthma	COPD
COPD	Neuromuscular disorders
Pneumonia	Drug toxicity
Pulmonary embolism	Head/neck injury
Pneumothorax	Life-threatening asthma

4.2 OXYGEN PRESCRIPTION

Indications

- $\downarrow$ SpO_2 (as measured by pulse oximetry)
- $\downarrow$ PaO_2 (as measured by ABG analysis)

Investigations

- Measure SpO_2 and PaO_2 in all breathless/acutely unwell patients
- Take ABG sample 30 min after every change to oxygen delivery

Management

- See Fig. 4.2

MICRO-facts

Hypoxia kills!
Target oxygen saturations:
- Normal adult: 94–98%
- Risk of hypercapnoea: 88–92%

Emergency and acute medicine

Emergency and acute medicine

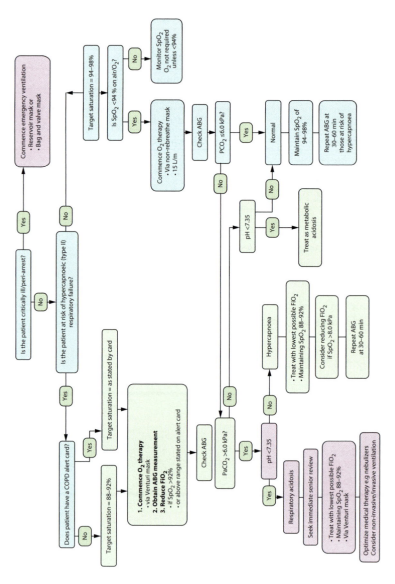

Fig. 4.2 Adapted BTS oxygen therapy guidelines.

4.3 ACUTE ASTHMA EXACERBATION: 'ASTHMA ATTACK'

Definition

- Acute onset worsening of patient's normal state, beyond day-to-day variation
- Severity determined by peak expiratory flow (PEF) as a percentage of normal

Clinical features

- See Fig. 4.3

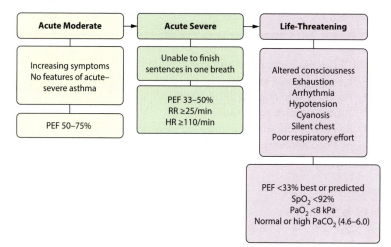

Fig. 4.3 Clinical features of asthma.

Investigations

- Peak expiratory flow (PEF):
  - Compare with patient's usual values from previous 2 years
  - If unavailable, use standard predicted values
  - Measure:
    - On admission
    - 30 min after treatment
    - According to response
- Pulse oximetry:
  - Monitor continuously
  - Ideal range = 94–98%

- Arterial blood gases:
  - Measure:
    - On admission
    - After 1 h: if patient deteriorates
    - After 4–6 h: with heart rate, potassium and glucose

MICRO-facts

Salbutamol may cause:
- **Tachycardia,** as it is a β2-adrenergic receptor agonist
- **Hypokalaemia**, as salbutamol drives potassium into cells
- **Hypoglycaemia**, as potassium is co-transported into cells with glucose

---

- Chest X-ray: not routine, but consider if:
  - Life-threatening asthma
  - Patient fails to respond to treatment
  - Patient requires ventilation
  - Any of the following are suspected following examination:
    - Pneumothorax
    - Consolidation

Management
- See Fig. 4.4

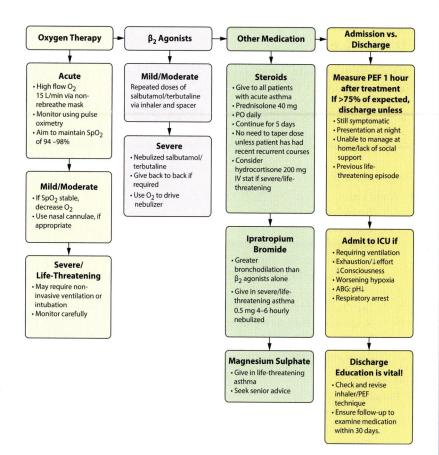

Fig. 4.4 Management of asthma.

4.4 EXACERBATION OF COPD

Definition

- Acute onset worsening of patient's normal state, beyond day-to-day variation

Aetiology

- Viral upper respiratory tract infection (URTI)
- Bacterial (LRTI)
- Non-infectious

> ## MICRO-facts
>
> **Non-infectious causes of exacerbations:**
> - Air pollution
> - Chronic heart failure
> - Pulmonary embolism
> - Myocardial infarction

Clinical features

- Symptoms:
  - Breathlessness
  - Cough
  - Increased sputum production or purulence
  - Decreased exercise tolerance
  - New onset or increased fluid retention
- Signs:
  - Increased respiratory rate
  - Respiratory distress, e.g. use of accessory muscles
  - New-onset cyanosis
  - Acute confusion

Investigations

- Bloods:
  - FBC: check for anaemia and raised white cell count
  - U&E
  - CRP: baseline measurement for monitoring
  - Blood cultures: if patient pyrexial
  - ABG: compare with previous, if possible
  - Theophylline level: if patient on theophylline on admission
- CXR:
  - To rule out pneumonia/pneumothorax
  - Hyperexpanded chest
  - Flat diaphragm
  - Barrel-shaped rib cage
- ECG:
  - To rule out myocardial infarction, arrhythmia and pulmonary embolism
- Sputum culture:
  - MC&S if purulent sputum
- Viral throat swab

Management

- See Fig. 4.5

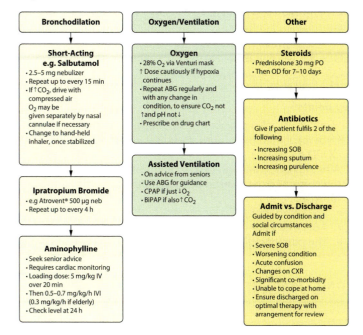

Bronchodilation

Short-Acting e.g. Salbutamol
- 2.5–5 mg nebulizer
- Repeat up to every 15 min
- If ↑CO_2, drive with compressed air O_2 may be given separately by nasal cannulae if necessary
- Change to hand-held inhaler, once stabilized

Ipratropium Bromide
- e.g Atrovent® 500 µg neb
- Repeat up to every 4 h

Aminophylline
- Seek senior advice
- Requires cardiac monitoring
- Loading dose: 5 mg/kg IV over 20 min
- Then 0.5–0.7 mg/kg/h IVI (0.3 mg/kg/h if elderly)
- Check level at 24 h

Oxygen/Ventilation

Oxygen
- 28% O_2 via Venturi mask
- ↑ Dose cautiously if hypoxia continues
- Repeat ABG regularly and with any change in condition, to ensure CO_2 not ↑and pH not ↓
- Prescribe on drug chart

Assisted Ventilation
- On advice from seniors
- Use ABG for guidance
- CPAP if just ↓O_2
- BiPAP if also↑CO_2

Other

Steroids
- Prednisolone 30 mg PO
- Then OD for 7–10 days

Antibiotics
Give if patient fulfils 2 of the following
- Increasing SOB
- Increasing sputum
- Increasing purulence

Admit vs. Discharge
Guided by condition and social circumstances
Admit if
- Severe SOB
- Worsening condition
- Acute confusion
- Changes on CXR
- Significant co-morbidity
- Unable to cope at home
- Ensure discharged on optimal therapy with arrangement for review

Fig. 4.5 Management of COPD.

MICRO-case

You are the foundation doctor in MAU and you have been asked to see a 60-year-old woman with known COPD who presented to the ED with severe shortness of breath. On initial assessment her initial ABG showed:

- pH = 7.37 (normal)
- PaO_2 = 7.5 kPa (hypoxaemia)
- $PaCO_2$ = 6.2 kPa (mild hypercapnoea)
- HCO_3^- = 35 (raised)

She was put on high-flow oxygen at a rate of 8 L/min; however, she is now drowsy and unwell. An ABG reading taken by your colleague 10 min ago shows:

- pH = 7.31 (acidosis)
- PaO_2 = 11
- $PaCO_2$ = 12 (hypercapnoea)
- HCO_3^- = 29

continued...

continued...

You immediately switch her oxygen to 24% via a venturi mask and perform a further ABG reading 30 min later, which gives the following results:

- pH = 7.35 (normal)
- PaO_2 = 8.5 kPa (hypoxaemia)
- $PaCO_2$ = 6.5 kPa (mild hypercapnoea)
- HCO_3^- = 33 (raised)

Key points:

- Hypoxia will kill a patient – do not hesitate when prescribing O_2.
- Hypercapnoea may occur with excessive oxygen in high-risk COPD patients.
- Aim to provide enough oxygen to maintain the patient's SpO_2 at the correct target level, in this case 88–92%.
- Monitor:
  - SpO_2 frequently
  - ABG every 30–60 min after every change to FiO_2
  - The patient's clinical condition: e.g. drowsiness/tiring easily

4.5 PNEUMONIA

Definition

- Acute infection of the lower respiratory tract, causing changes on chest X-ray

Aetiology

- Usually bacterial:
  - Streptococcus pneumoniae (50%)
  - Others, e.g. *Mycoplasma, Chlamydia, Legionella* spp.
- Viral, e.g. influenza virus A (5%)

Risk factors

- Advanced or very young age
- Immunocompromised
- Coexisting lung disease
- Smoking
- Vomiting (aspiration pneumonia)

Clinical features

- Lower respiratory tract symptoms:
  - SOB
  - Cough
  - Purulent sputum

- Wheeze
- Haemoptysis
- Pleuritic chest pain
- Systemic features:
  - ↑ RR/HR
  - Fever (>38°C)
  - Shivering
  - Confusion (especially elderly)
- On examination:
  - Dullness to percussion over affected area
  - ↓ Chest expansion on affected side
  - Bronchial breathing and coarse crackles on auscultation

Investigations

- Basic: regular SpO_2 monitoring (pulse oximetry)
- Bloods:
  - FBC (leukocytosis)
  - U&E (severity assessment)
  - CRP (monitor efficacy of treatment)
  - LFT
  - ABG (assess respiratory compromise)
- Calculate CURB65 score:
  - Severity assessment
- Microbiological (if severe or moderate CURB65 score):
  - Blood cultures (before commencing antibiotics)
  - Sputum sample: MC&S (moderate/producing sputum)
  - Bronchoalveolar lavage: MC&S (severe/unable to produce sputum)
- Specific tests:
  - Chest X-ray:
    - New focal consolidation (see Fig. 4.6)
  - Urine sample (if severe):
    - *S. pneumoniae* urine antigen test
    - Legionella urine antigen (if clear risk factors)

MICRO-facts

Legionella risk factors:

Water (e.g. air conditioning)
Age (elderly)
Immunocompromised
Lung disease
Smoker

Emergency and acute medicine

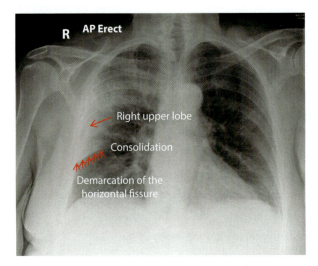

Fig. 4.6 Chest X-ray showing focal consolidation of right upper lobe pneumonia.

Management

- According to CURB65 severity assessment (Fig. 4.7)

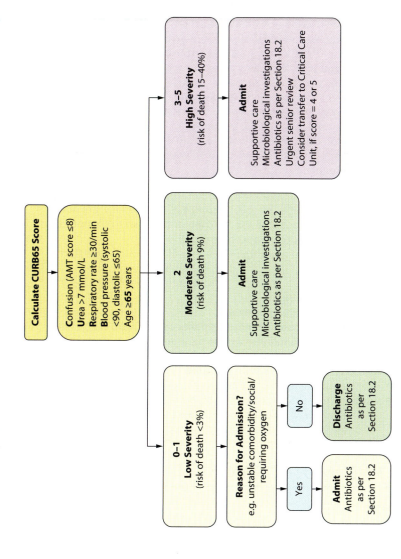

Calculate CURB65 Score

Confusion (AMT score ≤8)
Urea >7 mmol/L
Respiratory rate ≥30/min
Blood pressure (systolic <90, diastolic ≤65)
Age ≥65 years

0–1
Low Severity
(risk of death <3%)

Reason for Admission?
e.g. unstable comorbidity/social/
requiring oxygen

Yes → **Admit**
Antibiotics
as per
Section 18.2

No → **Discharge**
Antibiotics
as per
Section 18.2

2
Moderate Severity
(risk of death 9%)

Admit
Supportive care
Microbiological investigations
Antibiotics as per Section 18.2

3–5
High Severity
(risk of death 15–40%)

Admit
Supportive care
Microbiological investigations
Antibiotics as per Section 18.2
Urgent senior review
Consider transfer to Critical Care
Unit, if score = 4 or 5

Fig. 4.7 Management of pneumonia.

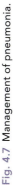

Emergency and acute medicine

MICRO-case

You are a junior doctor working nights in the ED and you have been called to see a 70-year-old man from a residential home. He is confused and suffers from type II diabetes mellitus. The paramedics explain that he has been increasingly confused and unwell over the past few days and is now dyspnoeic with a productive cough. On examination he has a blood pressure of 80/60 with a respiratory rate of 32 bpm. On auscultation of the lung bases, you notice coarse crackles at the left lung base. Blood tests show a raised white cell count and a raised CRP, but normal serum urea and glucose. A chest X-ray shows consolidation in the left lower lobe. You send blood cultures and a sputum sample for microscopy, culture and sensitivity before starting the gentleman on IV fluids and empirical antibiotic treatment for a community-acquired pneumonia. You calculate that he has a CURB65 score of 4, so you ask a senior member of staff to review him with you and discuss his case with the critical care team.

Key points:

- Always try to get a collateral history e.g. from family/care nurses.
  - If this is not possible e.g. at night, ensure that this is noted to be followed up the next morning.
- Always calculate a CURB65 score for patients with suspected pneumonia.
  - This man has a 'high risk' score and therefore has a 15–40% chance of dying.
  - He may require critical care.
- Always obtain baseline measurements of WCC and CRP, as this will allow staff to monitor a patient's response to treatment.
- An infection may alter a patient's glucose levels. Always check this in a patient with known diabetes.
- Start empirical antibiotic therapy as soon as possible.
- Always try to send sputum and blood culture samples for MC&S.
  - This will allow tailoring of antibiotic treatment if the patient does not respond to empirical therapy.

4.6 PNEUMOTHORAX

Definition

- Air in the pleural space

Clinical features

- General:
  - May be asymptomatic
  - Acute-onset SOB

- Acute-onset pleuritic chest pain
- ↓ Breath sounds
- Ipsilateral hyperresonant percussion note
- Ipsilateral ↓ chest expansion
- Primary spontaneous pneumothorax (PSP):
  - Healthy individuals
  - Tall
  - Male
- Secondary spontaneous pneumothorax (SSP):
  - Underlying lung disease
    - Asthma
    - Pneumonia
    - Abscess
    - Lung cancer
    - Emphysema
    - Smoker
- Tension pneumothorax:
  - As above, plus any of the following:
    - Severe respiratory distress
    - Hypotension
    - Tracheal deviation (to contralateral side)
    - Displaced apex beat
    - Distended neck veins

Investigations

- ABG:
  - To assess level of respiratory compromise
- CXR:
  - Is air present outside of the lung?
  - Measure distance between chest wall and lung

Management

- Follow flowchart in Fig. 4.8
- Traumatic or recurrent pneumothorax should always be referred to cardiothoracic surgery

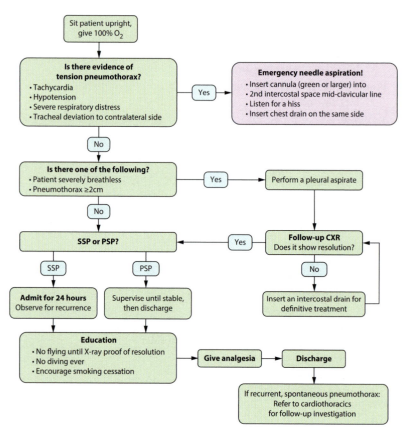

Fig. 4.8 Management of pneumothorax.

4.7 DEEP VEIN THROMBOSIS (DVT)

Definition

- A blood clot formed in the deep veins of the leg
- Most commonly:
  - Popliteal
  - Femoral
  - Iliac

Risk factors

- Virchow triad: is shown in Fig. 4.9.

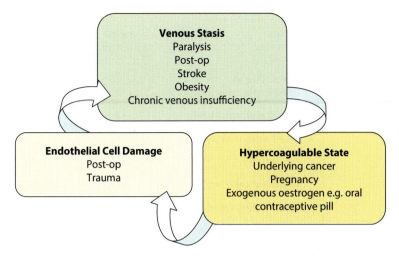

Venous Stasis
Paralysis
Post-op
Stroke
Obesity
Chronic venous insufficiency

Endothelial Cell Damage
Post-op
Trauma

Hypercoagulable State
Underlying cancer
Pregnancy
Exogenous oestrogen e.g. oral
contraceptive pill

Fig. 4.9 Virchow triad.

Clinical features

- Present in only 50% of cases:
    - Unilateral leg pain, improved with elevation
    - Unilateral leg swelling
    - Mild fever
    - Persistent tachycardia
    - Unilateral discolouration (rare)

Investigations

- Bloods:
    - FBC (thrombocytosis/polycythaemia)
    - Clotting screen (may need to commence anticoagulation)
    - U&E, LFT
- ECG: changes may be present if pulmonary embolism has occurred
- Clinical assessment: Wells criteria for deep vein thrombosis (see Fig. 4.10):

Management

- Treat PE, if present (see Section 4.8)
- Elevate affected limb
- Analgesia
- Further investigation, e.g. abdominal ultrasound if no clear risk factors present
- Graduated compression stockings to reduce the occurrence of post-thrombotic syndrome

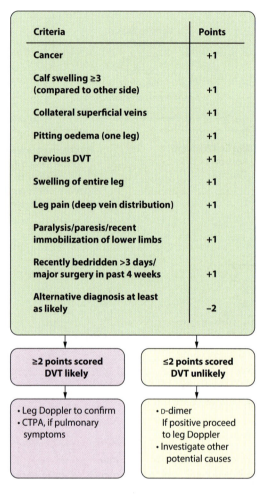

Criteria	Points
Cancer	+1
Calf swelling ≥3 (compared to other side)	+1
Collateral superficial veins	+1
Pitting oedema (one leg)	+1
Previous DVT	+1
Swelling of entire leg	+1
Leg pain (deep vein distribution)	+1
Paralysis/paresis/recent immobilization of lower limbs	+1
Recently bedridden >3 days/ major surgery in past 4 weeks	+1
Alternative diagnosis at least as likely	−2

≥2 points scored DVT likely
- Leg Doppler to confirm
- CTPA, if pulmonary symptoms

≤2 points scored DVT unlikely
- D-dimer If positive proceed to leg Doppler
- Investigate other potential causes

Fig. 4.10 Wells criteria for DVT.

- Low molecular weight heparin (LMWH):
  - If creatinine clearance <30, use unfractionated heparin
- Warfarin:
  - Target INR = 2.5 (±0.5)
  - Stop LMWH when INR is therapeutic on two consecutive readings
  - Treat for:
    - 6 weeks (calf vein thrombosis)
    - 3 months (proximal thrombosis, above peroneal)
    - ≥6 months/lifelong, if permanent risk factors or recurrence

> ## MICRO-facts
> Oral direct thrombin inhibitors and factor Xa inhibitors are currently under evaluation by NICE for treatment of DVT. They require no monitoring, are given as a single dose, but are not reversible.

> **MICRO-print**
> Catheter-directed thrombolysis is available in some centres for selected patients with ileofemoral DVT.

4.8 PULMONARY EMBOLISM (PE)

Definition

- Occlusion of an artery in the lung by an intravascular mass that has travelled through the bloodstream from a distant site

Aetiology

- Thromboembolic from DVT (90%)
- Other (these require treatment other than anticoagulation):
    - Fat: from a fracture
    - Air: from central venous catheterization
    - Amniotic fluid: during delivery
    - Septic e.g. from endocarditis

Clinical features

- Symptoms:
    - Breathlessness
    - Chest pain: usually pleuritic
    - Haemoptysis
    - Presyncope: feeling faint, dizzy
    - Syncope: collapse
    - Clinical signs of deep vein thrombosis (30%)
- Signs:
    - Tachycardia
    - Tachypnoea
    - Hypoxia
    - Haemodynamic compromise
    - Pyrexia
    - Pleural rub

Emergency and acute medicine

Investigations

- ABG: $\downarrow CO_2$/hypoxia
- ECG:
  - Sinus tachycardia (by far the most common ECG finding)
  - Right bundle branch block (RBBB)
  - Right axis deviation
  - $S_1Q_3T_3$ pattern (commonly learned, but rarely seen)

MICRO-print

The $S_1Q_3T_3$ pattern refers to:
- A large **S** wave in lead **1**
- A large **Q** wave in lead **3**
- An inverted **T** wave in lead **3**

Clinical assessment

- Wells criteria for pulmonary embolism: is shown in Fig. 4.11.

Criteria	Points
Clinically suspected DVT	+3
Alternative diagnosis less likely than PE	+3
Tachycardia	+1.5
Immobilization/surgery in past 4 weeks	+1.5
History of DVT or PE	+1.5
Haemoptysis	+1
Malignancy	+1

≥4 points scored PE likely
- Leg vein Doppler to confirm
- CTPA, if pulmonary symptoms

≤4 points scored PE unlikely
- Use D-dimer to further rule out
- Investigate other potential causes

Fig. 4.11 Wells criteria for PE.

Management

- Oxygen if hypoxic
- Analgesia
- Check troponin and echocardiogram to assess for signs of right heart strain
- Consider thrombolysis: if CTPA shows massive PE + signs of haemodynamic compromise:
    - Alteplase, 50 mg bolus
    - Check for contraindications before administration (as for STEMI; see Section 3.1)
- LMWH or unfractionated heparin: see DVT section for doses (Section 9.1)
- Warfarin/direct thrombin inhibitor:
    - Start once venous thromboembolism confirmed
    - See DVT section for doses (Section 4.7)
- Consider inferior vena cava filter if anticoagulation contraindicated

---

MICRO-print

Surgical embolectomy and catheter-directed thrombolysis may be considered in selected patients in some centres.

4.9 PLEURAL EFFUSION

Definition

- Excess fluid in the pleural space
- Approximately 300 mL of fluid needs to be present before clinically detectable

Aetiology

- Divided into two groups:
    - Exudates
    - Transudates
- Determined by Light's criteria for an exudate
- For simplicity, fluid protein levels are often used in isolation assuming a normal blood protein level
    - Fluid protein >30 g/L indicates exudate
    - Fluid protein <30 g/L indicates transudate
- Other indicators:
    - Transudate usually bilateral, exudate usually unilateral
    - ↑ WCC indicates exudates

Clinical features

- Symptoms:
    - May be asymptomatic
    - Pleuritic chest pain

- Breathlessness
- Significant hypoxia/haemodynamic compromise if severe
- Systemic features of associated disease:
  - Signs of chronic liver disease
  - History of previous malignancy
  - Recent pneumonic symptoms
- Signs:
  - Decreased chest expansion
  - Stoney dull percussion note
  - Decreased breath sounds on the affected side
  - Tracheal deviation away from affected side, if large

Investigations

- Chest X-ray
- Ultrasound can help identify the presence of fluid and guide aspiration
- Diagnostic tap using ultrasound guidance
  - 30 mL aspirated sent for MC+S, cytology and biochemical (see Table 4.2)

Table 4.2 **Diagnosis of pleural effusion**

TRANSUDATE	EXUDATE
PROTEIN CONTENT <30 G/L	PROTEIN CONTENT >30 G/L
• Heart failure by far the most common cause • Liver failure • Renal failure • Hypoalbuminaemia • Hypothyroidism • Sarcoidosis • Meig's syndrome Right pleural effusion and ovarian fibroma • Pulmonary embolus (usually an exudate)	• Pneumonia – parapneumonic effusion • Empyema • Malignancy – local or metastatic • Tuberculosis • Pulmonary embolus • Pancreatitis • Connective tissue disorders • Drug-induced, e.g. amiodarone • Chylothorax • Post-coronary artery bypass surgery

Management

- Dependent on the underlying cause
- Consider drainage if patient symptomatic or empyema suspected
  - Requires insertion of intercostal drain, usually under ultrasound or CT guidance
  - Avoid rapid drainage which can precipitate pulmonary oedema (<2 L/4 h)
- Consider talc pleuradesis in malignancy and recurrent effusion
  - Inserted via intercostal (approx 60% success rate)

- Palliative aspiration via a large-bore cannula
  - Associated with high rate of recurrence at 1 month, so best avoided unless very short life expectancy
  - Performed 2 L at a time, ideally under ultrasound guidance
- Surgery may be considered for recurrent effusions or increasing pleural thickening

---

MICRO-print

Thoracoscopy may be performed under sedation for visual assessment of the pleura, complete removal of fluid, pleural biopsy and talc pleuridesis. Discuss with senior colleagues.

CT thorax can help aid diagnosis of underlying disease and guide pleural biopsy if thoracoscopy not available or appropriate.

5 Gastroenterology

5.1 UPPER GASTROINTESTINAL (GI) BLEED

Definition
- Bleeding originating proximal to the ligament of Treitz (oesophagus, stomach and duodenum)

Aetiology
- Common:
  - Peptic/duodenal ulcer
  - Oesophagitis/gastritis/duodenitis
  - Mallory-Weiss tear
  - Oesophageal varices
  - Swallowed blood
- Less common:
  - Upper GI malignancy (may also present with melaena)
  - Coagulation abnormalities
  - Vascular malformation angiodysplasia
  - Gastric antral vascular ectasia (GAVE)
  - Hereditary haemorrhagic telangiectasia
  - Aorto-enteric fistula

Risk factors
- Previous ulcer
- Chronic alcohol consumption
- ↑ Age
- Acute illness
- *H. pylori* infection
- Drugs:
  - NSAIDs
  - Aspirin
  - Anticoagulants
  - Thrombolytics

- Corticosteroids
- SSRIs

Clinical features

- See Table 5.1
- Haematemesis: vomited blood
  - Bright red
  - Dark clots
  - Coffee grounds
- Melaena: Black 'tarry' stools
- Dark red blood on PR
- Epigastric pain
- Stigmata of chronic liver disease:
  - Jaundice
  - Clubbing
  - Caput medusae
  - Spider naevi
  - Ascites
- Chest pain/retrosternal pain
- Sweating and palpitations
- Hypovolaemia:
  - Postural dizziness
  - Confusion
  - Shock
  - Collapse

> **MICRO-facts**
>
> Upper GI bleed can present with fresh PR blood if very severe.

Table 5.1 **Clinical features of upper GI bleed according to cause**

AETIOLOGY	FEATURES
Peptic ulceration	• Epigastric/chest pain • Heartburn • Melaena • Past medical history: NSAIDs, alcohol, previous ulcer
Oesophagitis/gastritis	• Heartburn • Epigastric tenderness • Past medical history: NSAIDs, alcohol

(Continued)

Table 5.1 *(Continued)* **Clinical features of upper GI bleed according to cause**

AETIOLOGY	FEATURES
Oesophageal varices	• Frank haematemesis • Epigastric pain • Signs of chronic liver disease • Chronic alcohol excess • Known varices
Mallory-Weiss tear	• Normal colour • Forceful vomit prior to haematemesis • Epigastric tenderness
Swallowed blood	• Epistaxis • Haemoptysis

Assessing severity

- Indicators of severity:
    - Age >60
    - BP <100
    - HR >120 (may not be elevated if patient taking beta-blockers)
    - Chronic liver disease
    - Other comorbidities: cardiac, renal, respiratory
    - Decreased consciousness
    - ↓ Urine output
    - Pallor
    - Cold peripheries

Investigations

- Blood tests:
    - FBC: Hb may be ↓ or normal
    - U&E: ↑ urea out of proportion to creatinine
    - LFT: liver failure may lead to clotting abnormalities and/or varices
    - Clotting
    - Group and save (if mild bleed)
    - Cross-match 6 units (if severe bleed)
- CXR: May show pleural effusion
- Oesophageoduodenoscopy (OGD):
    - Severe bleed/shock: perform within 4 h, but fluid resuscitate first
    - Mild bleed: perform within 24 h

Management of acute upper GI bleed

- See Fig. 5.1

Emergency and acute medicine

Further management

- Proton pump inhibitor (PPI):
  - 72 h IV infusion reduces the risk of re-bleeding in endoscopically confirmed lesions
- Assess risk of re-bleeding:
  - See Rockall score (Table 5.2)
- If known varices, IV antibiotics e.g. co-amoxiclav and terlipressin
- Keep nil by mouth for 24 h
- Correct coagulation abnormalities
- Monitoring:
  - Hourly if unstable, 4 hourly if stable: vital signs, urine output
  - Regular bloods: FBC, U&E and LFT; clotting if abnormal, or massive transfusion

---

MICRO-facts

Giving a PPI after endoscopy reduces the risk of re-bleeding.

Signs of re-bleed

- ↑ HR
- ↓ Urine output
- Haematemesis, or continuing melaena
- ↓ BP: may be a late sign
- ↓ Level of consciousness
- Falling Hb/climbing urea
- Add the scores for each line to produce a total score
- Score 0–1: low risk of re-bleed and may be suitable for early discharge
- Score ≥5: high risk of re-bleed (25%) and closely monitor patient, consider HDU

MICRO-reference

Scottish Intercollegiate Guidelines Network (SIGN) – Acute Upper and Lower GI Bleeding, http://www.sign.ac.uk/pdf/sign105.pdf

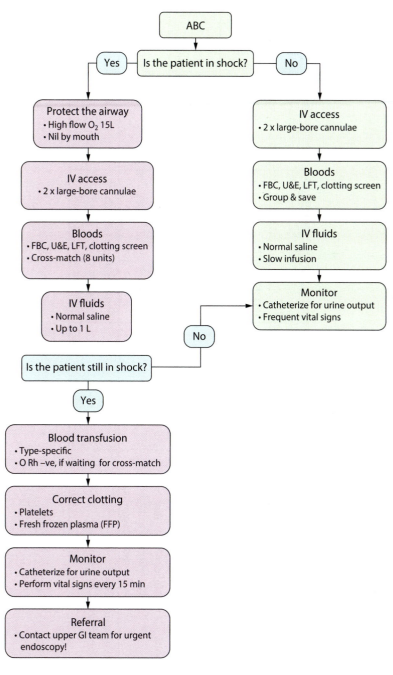

Fig. 5.1 Management of upper GI bleeds.

Emergency and acute medicine

Table 5.2 Rockall scoring

VARIABLE	0	1	2	3
Age	<60 years	60–79 years	>80 years	
Shock	Not shocked SBP >100 mmHg Pulse <100 bpm	Tachycardic SBP >100 mmHg Pulse >100 bpm	Hypotension SBP <100 mmHg	
Comorbidity	None		Cardiac failure IHD Any major comorbidity	Renal failure Liver failure Disseminated malignancy
Diagnosis	Mallory-Weiss tear No lesion identified No recent haemorrhage	All other diagnoses	Malignancy of upper GI tract	
Major stigmata of haemorrhage	None Dark spot only		Blood in upper GI tract Adherent clot Visible or spurting vessel	

5.2 OESOPHAGEAL VARICES

Definition
- Abnormally distended veins in the oeseophagus, which are at risk of rupture; bleeding is characteristically severe

Clinical features
- Known varices
- History of alcohol abuse
- Signs of chronic liver disease:
  - Hepatomegaly (liver may also be cirrhotic and small)
  - Splenomegaly
  - Ascites
  - Encephalopathy – confusion, liver flap

Management
- ABC
- Involve seniors early
- Urgent cross-match: 6–8 units of blood or transfuse O-ve blood
- Correct clotting: vitamin K, fresh frozen plasma (FFP)
- IV terlipressin and antibiotics
- Discuss with on-call endoscopist: may need emergency endoscopic banding
- Balloon tamponade:
  - Uncontrolled/life-threatening bleeding
  - Needs anaesthetic review for consideration of possible intubation for airway protection
  - Seek senior/radiology advice

MICRO-facts

Attempt resuscitation before endoscopy.

MICRO-case

A 56-year-old man attends the ED after two episodes of melaena and vomiting fresh blood. During initial assessment by the junior doctor, the patient has a further fresh haematemesis and becomes haemodynamically unstable. He is resuscitated with two fluid boluses of 500 mL colloid over 30 min which restores his blood pressure. Once he is haemodynamically stable, the junior doctor continues with the assessment and learns that the patient has a history of heavy alcohol consumption and recent

continued...

continued...

ibuprofen use. The doctor requests for urgent upper GI endoscopy for a possible peptic ulcer or oeesophageal variceal bleed.

- Resuscitation with fluid and/or blood (no consensus on colloid vs crystalloid).
- Acute GI bleeds do not always cause a drop in Hb immediately; therefore normal Hb does not exclude a bleed.
- Gain IV access for FBC, clotting, G + S and cross-match for 4–6 units of blood if moderate/severe bleeding.
- Raised urea and normal creatinine are the result of absorption of protein from digested blood.
- The patient should undergo endoscopy to identify the cause of bleeding.
- The risk of re-bleed should be calculated and prevented with referral to the surgeons if the patient is considered high risk.

5.3 LOWER GI BLEED

Definition

- Bleeding originating from the small bowel and colon

Aetiology

- See Table 5.3

Table 5.3 **Causes and clinical features of lower GI bleeds**

CAUSES	CLINICAL FEATURES
Diverticular disease	• Abdominal pain • Fever: diverticulitis • Change in bowel habit • Tender/peritonism • PR: blood
Colorectal polyps	• Intermittent abdominal pain • Change in bowel habit • Tenesmus • Weight loss • PR: blood and palpable mass • Family history
Colorectal cancer	• Change in bowel habit • Weight loss • Abdominal pain • PR: blood, mucus, palpable mass

(Continued)

Table 5.3 *(Continued)* **Causes and clinical features of lower GI bleeds**

CAUSES	CLINICAL FEATURES
Inflammatory bowel disease (IBD)	• Abdominal pain • Diarrhoea • Weight loss • Extra intestinal features: mouth ulcers, erythema nodosum, anterior uveitis • Fever • Tenesmus and urgency • PR: blood, mucus
Haemorrhoids	• Painless • Fresh blood on toilet paper • Perianal itch • Constipation • PR: not always visible or palpable • Prolapse through anus
Anal fissure	• Pain • Fresh blood on toilet paper • Constipation • PR: tear, pain ++
Bowel ischaemia	• Severe abdominal pain • Shocked • Absence of bowel sounds • Past medical history: previous arterial disease, atrial fibrillation
Upper GI bleed	• PR: melaena • Epigastric pain • Signs of liver disease

Investigations

- Isolated episode in a person <45 years of age:
    - PR
    - Proctoscopy
    - >45 years/family history/known inflammatory bowel disease
    - PR: blood, palpable mass
    - Blood tests: FBC, U&E, LFT, clotting, glucose, group and save
    - Proctoscopy: haemorrhoids
    - OGD: exclude upper GI bleed
    - Sigmoidoscopy/colonoscopy: visualization ± biopsy of inflammatory bowel disease and colonic cancer

Emergency and acute medicine

- CT abdomen: ischaemic colitis
- CT angiography: unidentified source of continuous bleeding, and possible embolization

Management

- See Table 5.4

Table 5.4 **Management of lower GI bleed**

SEVERITY	MANAGEMENT
Mild	• NBM • IV access + fluids • Obs – HR, BP, UO • Reassess if further bleeding, most resolve spontaneously
Moderate	• Resuscitate with colloids/blood until stable • Insert catheter • Fluid balance • Senior review
Severe	• Treat as upper GI bleed

MICRO-facts

The majority of lower GI bleeds will resolve spontaneously without specific treatment.

5.4 INFLAMMATORY BOWEL DISEASE

Definition

- A group of conditions characterized by intestinal inflammation
  - Ulcerative colitis: regional
  - Crohn's disease: can affect any part of the GI tract ('mouth to anus')

Clinical features

- See Table 5.5

Table 5.5 **Comparison of ulcerative colitis and Crohn's disease**

	ULCERATIVE COLITIS	CROHN'S DISEASE
Clinical features	• Bloody diarrhoea • Colicky abdominal pain • Urgency • Tenesmus • Fever	• Abdominal pain • Diarrhoea • Weight loss • Malaise • Anorexia • Fever

Extraintestinal features

- Anterior uveitis
- Seronegative arthropathies: ankylosing spondylitis
- Erythema nodosum

Features of severe episode

- >6 Bloody stools/day
- Systemically unwell
- Hb <10 g/dL
- Toxic dilatation (colon >6 cm on imaging; see Fig. 5.2)
- Hypoalbuminaemia

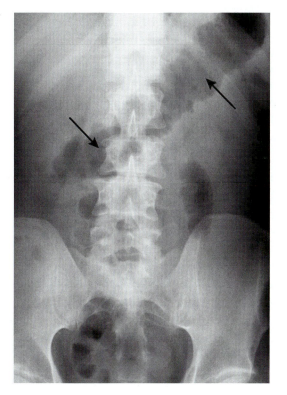

Fig. 5.2 AXR of toxic megacolon.

Investigations

- Bloods:
  - FBC
    - Hb: may be low if chronic bleeding
    - WCC: raised in inflammation and infection

- U&E: urea may be raised in active bleeding
- Inflammatory markers (CRP and ESR): raised
- Clotting profile: can be deranged if profuse bleeding
- LFTs (albumin)
- Stool culture to rule out infection, particularly *Clostridium difficile*
- Rigid sigmoidoscopy: inflamed mucosa, may show bleeding
- Abdominal plain radiograph: thumbprinting of intestinal lining

Management

- IV fluids
- IV steroids: 100 mg hydrocortisone QDS
- Antibiotics: metronidazole 400 mg IV/oral TDS
- Rectal steroid foam or mesalazine, if distal disease
- Referral to surgery if:
  - Perforation
  - Haemorrhage
  - Toxic dilatation
  - Patient on cytotoxic drugs: mesalazine or azathioprine
- Nil by mouth

MICRO-reference

British Society of Gastroenterology – Guidelines for the Management of Inflammatory Bowel Disease, http://www.bsg.org.uk/clinical-guidelines/ibd/guidelines-for-the-management-of-inflammatory.html

---

5.5 DIARRHOEA

MICRO-facts

In acute diarrhoea ± vomiting, suspect gastroenteritis (Section 18.3).

Definition

- 3 or more loose stools/day

Aetiology

- Infective (see Chapter 18, Infectious Diseases)
- Non-infective:
  - UC
  - Crohn's disease
  - Colorectal cancer

- Colonic polyps
- Pseudomembranous colitis
- Ischaemic colitis
- IBS
- Diverticulitis
- Pancreatitis or pancreatic insufficiency
- Overflow diarrhoea
- Non-gastrointestinal causes:
  - Antibiotics
  - Alcohol
  - Lactose intolerance
  - Drugs (e.g. PPI)
  - Laxative abuse
  - Thyrotoxicosis
  - Autonomic neuropathy
  - Addison's disease

MICRO-facts

Key points in a history of diarrhoea

- Travel
- Diet
- Contact
- Recent antibiotics or laxatives

Clinical features

- Weight loss
- Clubbing: IBD, cirrhosis, chronic alcoholism (pancreatic insufficiency)
- Anaemia: IBD
- Mouth ulcers
- Rash: erythema nodosum
- Abdominal mass
- Goitre: thyrotoxicosis
- PR exam: mass, impacted stool, bleeding
- Dehydrated: dry mucous membranes, skin turgor
- Features of malabsorption e.g. B_{12} deficiency

Investigations

- Bloods:
  - FBC: Hb (anaemia), WCC (infection, inflammatory)
  - U&E: urea and creatinine (renal function, dehydration)

- Inflammatory markers: ESR, CRP (raised in infection and IBD)
- Thyroid function tests: diarrhoea in hyperthyroidism
- Group and save
- Stool sample: MC&S
- Sigmoidoscopy/colonoscopy

Management

- IV fluids
- Replace electrolytes
- Treat cause

> ### MICRO-facts
>
> In gastroenteritis do not give antibiotics unless systemically unwell. There is no evidence that it is effective and increases risk of *Clostridium difficile* infection.

5.6 ACUTE LIVER FAILURE

Definition

- Potentially reversible severe liver injury with onset of hepatic encephalopathy within 8 weeks of symptoms

Aetiology

- Paracetamol overdose
- Drug reactions e.g. NSAID, rifampicin, herbal remedies
- Viral hepatitis: hepatitis A, C and E
- Other infections:
  - Epstein-Barr virus
  - Cytomegalovirus
- Autoimmune
- Toxins: poisonous mushrooms (*Amanita phalloides*)
- Malignancy: primary, secondary
- Budd-Chiari syndrome
- Vascular/ischaemia
- Pregnancy: HELLP syndrome
- Other

Investigations

- Blood tests:
  - FBC
  - U&E
  - Glucose

  - Clotting screen
  - LFTs
  - Serum lactate
  - Bilirubin
  - Blood group and cross-match
  - ABG
  - Plasma ammonia
- Diagnostic tests:
  - Viral serology (including HIV)
  - Autoimmune screen
  - Paracetamol levels/urine toxicology screen
  - Blood tests for haemachromatosis, Wilson's and alpha-1-antitripsin if clinically indicated
- Bacteriology:
  - Blood cultures
  - Urine: dipstick/MC&S
  - Sputum culture
  - Throat swabs: MC&S
- USS: Liver with Doppler
- Chest radiograph
- EEG (rarely): hepatic encephalopathy
- Liver biopsy

ACUTE-ON-CHRONIC LIVER FAILURE

Aetiology

- Infection
- Acute GI haemorrhage
- Hepatotoxic injury
- Drugs
- Constipation
- Metabolic disturbance
- Surgery
- Acute (on chronic) increase in alcohol intake

Clinical features

- Symptoms:
  - Fatigue
  - Nausea/vomiting
  - Loss of appetite
  - Weight loss
  - Pruritis
  - Abdominal pain
  - Excessive sleepiness/confusion

- Social history:
  - Foreign travel
  - Blood transfusions: date of transfusion important i.e. prior to early 1990s
  - Sexual contacts
  - Occupation
  - Body piercing, tattoos
- Alcohol intake
- Drug history: recreational/prescription
- Herbal medicine
- Toxin ingestion
  - Poisonous mushrooms
  - Solvents
- Examination: (see Fig. 5.3)

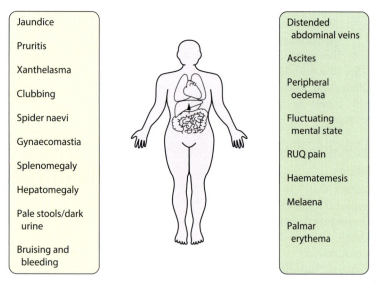

Jaundice	Distended abdominal veins
Pruritis	Ascites
Xanthelasma	Peripheral oedema
Clubbing	Fluctuating mental state
Spider naevi	RUQ pain
Gynaecomastia	Haematemesis
Splenomegaly	Melaena
Hepatomegaly	Palmar erythema
Pale stools/dark urine	
Bruising and bleeding	

Fig. 5.3 Examination findings in acute (on chronic) liver failure.

Management

- Consider HDU or ICU transfer
  - Nil by mouth if conscious level depressed
  - Catheterize and monitor hourly output
  - Treat alcohol withdrawal with a reducing regime of benzodiazepines
  - Correct electrolyte abnormalities
  - Treat cerebral oedema: mannitol
  - PPI (to reduce the risk of haemorrhagic gastritis

- Coagulopathy: vitamin K 10 mg IV, for 3 days. Consider FFP only if considering invasive procedure, or actively bleeding
- Hypoglycaemia: IV glucose
- Parenteral vitamins if alcohol dependent to reduce the risk of Wernicke's encephalopathy
- If requiring IV fluids avoid excessive normal saline as may make ascites worse
- Infection prophylaxis: broad spectrum antibiotics
- Acute renal failure/hepatorenal syndrome: fluid replacement, haemodialysis
- N-acetylcysteine, early use may prevent progression of encephalopathy, even in liver failure not associated with paracetamol toxicity
- Ascites: fluid restriction, low salt, daily weights, diuretics
- Nutritional support
- Treat underlying cause
- Patient may need transfer to a liver unit, or consideration for transplant; begin discussion with liver team early (see Table 5.6)

Table 5.6 **Kings' College criteria for transplant in acute liver failure**

Paracetamol	Arterial pH <7.3	• Or all three of:
		  • PT >100 s
		  • Creat >300 µmol/L
		  • Grade III or IV encephalopathy

Non-paracetamol	PT >100 s
	INR >6.7
		• Or any three of:
		  • Aetiology – drug reaction/seronegative hepatitis
		  • Age <10 years, >40 years
		  • PT >50, INR >4.0
		  • Serum bilirubin >300 µmol/L

5.7 HEPATIC ENCEPHALOPATHY

Definition

- Neuropsychiatric disturbance of cognitive function in a patient with liver disease

Clinical features

- ↑ Confusion: exclude other causes first
- Asterixis: liver flap
- Abnormal EEG
- ↑ Serum ammonia

MICRO-facts

Exclude other more common causes of ↑ confusion:

- Sepsis
- Metabolic disturbance
- Seizures

Investigations

- Bloods:
    - FBC: macrocytic anaemia
    - U&Es: low sodium and potassium
    - LFTs: deranged ALT, AST, GGT, ALP indicating hepatic failure; raised bilirubin
    - Clotting screen: deranged prothrombin time
    - Serum ammonia: raised
- CT head: cerebral oedema; to exclude other pathology
- EEG: high-amplitude, low-frequency waves and triphasic waves

Management

- May require ventilatory support
- Head elevated to 30°
- Treat cause:
    - GI bleed: see upper GI bleed (Chapter 5)
    - Infections: see empirical antibiotics doses (Section 18.2)
    - Renal failure (Section 8.1)
    - Electrolyte abnormalities (Section 7.4)
- Protein restriction: to decrease ammonia
- Lactulose: to reduce ammonia reabsorption and increase gut transit
- Nutritional support: NG tube or parenteral feed
- Avoid certain medications (see MICRO-fact)

MICRO-facts

Use the following with caution in patients with liver failure:

- Opiates
- Diuretics
- Oral hypoglycaemics e.g. metformin
- Warfarin
- Benzodiazepines

Complications

- Cerebral oedema
- Multi-organ failure:
  - Heart failure
  - Renal failure
- Sepsis
- Permanent neurological dysfunction
- Irreversible coma

5.8 ALCOHOL WITHDRAWAL SYNDROME

See Chapter 19, Psychiatry, for further information.

Definition

- A combination of central nervous system-mediated symptoms experienced following acute reduction or cessation of alcohol consumption, after chronic excessive intake

Aetiology

- Usually commences within 10–72 h
- Consider in all patients with new-onset confusion within 3 days of admission
- May occur in anybody consuming >8 units per day

Clinical features

- Tachycardia
- Tremor
- Sweating
- Agitation/confusion
- Headache
- Nausea and vomiting
- Seizures, which can result in death
- Hallucinations; delirium tremens
  - Visual e.g. small animals
  - Tactile e.g. insects on skin

Investigation

- Alcohol history – including collateral history
- Routinely clarify and document alcohol intake with every patient admitted to hospital
- Check glucose
- U&E, LFT, FBC, clotting

- Infection screen
- CT head if recent head injury or localizing neurology
- Consider non-invasive liver screen including an ultrasound if has not been investigated previously

Management

- Regular benzodiazepines e.g. chlordiazepoxide 15–30 mg QDS, or lorazepam if significant liver impairment.
- Also prescribe extra PRN for breakthrough symptoms.
- Reducing regime over 7–10 days.
- Haloperidol can also be used in conjunction with benzodiazepines if hallucinations predominate.
- Vitamins to prevent Wernicke's encephalopathy e.g. Pabrinex 2 ampules IV TDS for 3 days. Continue oral vitamins long term.
- Oral PPI.
- Most seizures are self-terminating, but may require treatment (see Section 6.3).
- Dietician review and nutritional supplements.
- Antiemetics.
- Aggressive treatment of infection.
- Review for signs of hepatic encephalopathy regularly.
- Occasionally may require HDU admission for sedation.
- Review by alcohol liaison nurses, to help patients abstain and provide support following discharge.

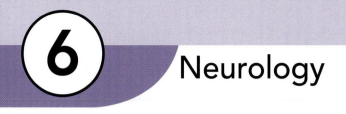

Neurology

6.1 STROKE

Definition
- Neurological deficit of cerebrovascular cause that persists beyond 24 h or is interrupted by death within 24 h

Epidemiology
- Age ≥55
- Those of African-American origin are at increased risk
- Male ≥ female

Risk factors
- Family history of stroke/transient ischaemic attack (TIA)
- Hypertension
- Diabetes
- Smoking
- Atrial fibrillation
- Hypercholesterolaemia
- Others include migraine, obstructive sleep apnoea

Pathophysiology
- Ischaemic:
  - 80%
  - Focal ischaemia leading to cerebral infarction
- Haemorrhagic:
  - 20%
  - Spontaneous bleeding into brain tissue
  - Includes:
    - Intracranial haemorrhage (90%)
    - Sub-arachnoid haemorrhage (10%)

Clinical features

- Numbness
- Weakness
- Paralysis
- Slurred speech
- Blurred vision
- Sudden-onset monocular visual loss (amaurosis fugax)
- Confusion
- ↓ Level of consciousness
- Severe headache

> **MICRO-facts**
>
> FAST stroke recognition:
>
> **F**ace: Is it drooped on one side/can they smile?
> **A**rms: Can they raise both and hold them up?
> **S**peech: Is it slurred?
> **T**ime: Diagnose and treat as soon as possible.

ISCHAEMIC VS. HAEMORRHAGIC STROKE

Clinical features

- See Table 6.1

Table 6.1 **Clinical features of ischaemic and haemorrhagic stroke**

FACTOR	ISCHAEMIC	HAEMORRHAGIC
Hypertension	Often present	Usually present
Preceding TIA?	30% of cases	No
Course	Usually static	Rapidly progressive
Increased ICP?	No	Yes
CT scan result	Normal, or consistent with infarct	Shows blood

Emergency and acute medicine

Diagnosis

Rule Out Stroke In the Emergency Room tool (ROSIER)

Has there been

- Loss of consciousness or syncope?   Yes (−1)   No (0)
- Seizure activity?   Yes (−1)   No (0)

Is there new onset (or on waking from sleep)

- Asymmetric facial weakness?   Yes (+1)   No (0)
- Asymmetric arm weakness?   Yes (+1)   No (0)
- Asymmetric leg weakness?   Yes (+1)   No (0)
- Speech disturbance?   Yes (+1)   No (0)
- Visual field defect?   Yes (+1)   No (0)

Score >0 Stroke = high probability
Score ≤0 Stroke = low probability, but not excluded

Fig. 6.1 Rule out stroke in the emergency room (ROSIER) tool.

Investigations

- Bloods:
    - Full blood count
    - Urea and electrolytes
    - Blood glucose
    - Clotting screen
- Imaging: CT head, non-contrast: check for haemorrhage or ischaemia
- ECG: rule out atrial fibrillation or acute myocardial infarction as source of emboli
- Infection screen: infection can often precipitate worsening of previous stroke symptoms

Management

• See Fig. 6.2

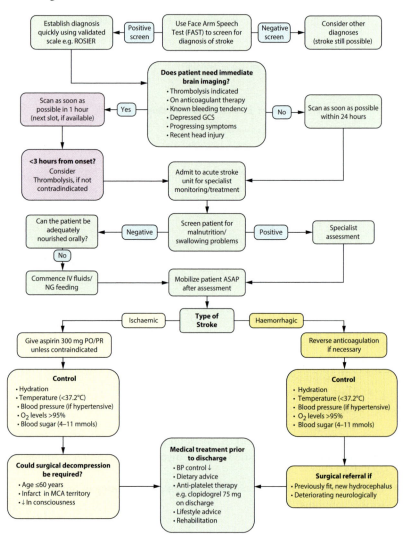

Fig. 6.2 Stroke management algorithm.

6.2 TRANSIENT ISCHAEMIC ATTACK

Definition

- Neurological dysfunction caused by a disruption in cerebral blood flow which lasts less than 24 h

> ### MICRO-facts
>
> 10–15% will go on to develop infarction within 3 months of initial TIA. Use ABCD^2 score for risk assessment.

Clinical features

- See 'Stroke' (Section 6.1) for signs and symptoms
- Symptoms resolve within minutes or a few hours
- Persistent neurological dysfunction? Treat as a stroke

Management

- See Figs. 6.3 and 6.4

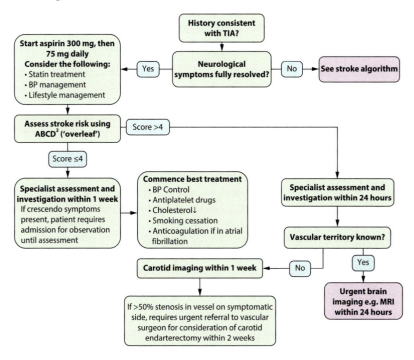

Fig. 6.3 Management of transient ischaemic attack.

Emergency and acute medicine

Stroke risk assessment

ABCD^2 Scale for TIA Assessment

Age >60 years	+1
Blood pressure >140/90 mm/Hg	+1
Clinical features	
• Unilateral weakness	+2
• Speech disturbance without weakness	+1
• Other	0
Duration	
• >60 minutes	+2
• 10–60 minutes	+1
• <10 minutes	0
Diabetes	+1

Risk of stroke at two days*

0–3 points = 1%
4–5 points = 4%
6–7 points = 8%

*Higher if more than one episode in one week

Fig. 6.4 ABCD^2 stroke risk assessment tool.

MICRO-case

A 60-year-old man presents to the ED complaining of weakness. He explains that he was trying to play his violin, but was unable to hold his bow with his right arm. His symptoms lasted approximately 1 h. He presents with no other symptoms. His blood pressure is 150/90 and his pulse is 65 bpm. An ECG shows sinus rhythm. On examination, he has no neurological deficit. You suspect that he has suffered a TIA, so you immediately give him 300 mg of aspirin. You calculate his ABCD^2 score to be 6, giving him a stroke risk of 8% at 2 days. You therefore commence treatment with a statin. You also arrange for him to see a stroke specialist and to undergo carotid imaging in a few days' time.

Key points:
- Patients often present with subtle symptoms, such as loss of function.
- Always calculate ABCD^2 stroke risk in any patient with TIA.

continued...

continued…

- Stroke risk is increased if a patient has had more than one episode.
- Patients with TIA must be seen by a specialist for investigation and treatment.
- If the vascular territory of the TIA is not known, carotid imaging must be performed within 1 week.

6.3 SEIZURES AND STATUS EPILEPTICUS

Definitions

- Seizure:
  - A sudden attack caused by abnormal electrical discharges within the brain, characterized by:
    - Convulsions
    - Sensory disturbances
    - Loss of consciousness
- Status epilepticus:
  - Single prolonged seizure
  - A series of seizures without intervening full recovery of consciousness

Aetiology

- Primary seizure disorder e.g. epilepsy
- Trauma
- Non-epileptic seizure disorder
- Intracranial haemorrhage
- Structural abnormality e.g. infarct, neoplasia
- Infection e.g. encephalitis
- Toxins/drugs
- Alcohol withdrawal
- Pregnancy
- Hypoxia
- Metabolic:
  - Hyper/hypoglycaemia
  - Hyper/hyponatraemia
  - Hypocalcaemia
  - Hypomagnesaemia
  - Uraemia

MICRO-facts

It is invaluable to take an additional history from a witness of the episode.

Emergency and acute medicine

Clinical features

- Preceding aura
- Rapid onset
- Loss of bladder/bowel control
- Tongue biting
- Physical injury:
  - Tongue laceration
  - Head/spine injuries from fall
  - Aspiration

Investigations

- Initial: blood glucose level (blood glucose meter)
- Bloods:
  - FBC
  - U&E
  - Drug levels
  - Toxicology screen
  - Blood cultures
- ECG
- Cranial imaging:
  - Emergency CT if any of the following:
    - Head trauma
    - Focal neurology
    - Bleeding disorder
    - Prolonged post-ictal period

Management

- Follow steps in Fig. 6.5
- If alcohol withdrawal suspected:
  - IV Pabrinex® (see Section 19.5)
  - If overdose/poisoning suspected: (see Section 10)
  - If pregnant: consider pre-eclampsia (see Section 15.10)

Further management

- Patients with known epilepsy: investigate cause of poor seizure control:
  - Check anticonvulsant levels
  - Screen for infection or electrolyte abnormality
  - Assess for adherence and educate as required
- New onset seizures: investigate underlying cause:
  - Refer to neurology
  - Organize CT or MRI to exclude structural lesion

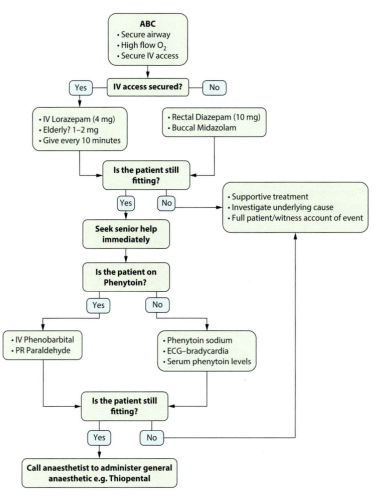

Fig. 6.5 Management of seizures.

6.4 TRANSIENT LOSS OF CONSCIOUSNESS (SYNCOPE)

Definition

- Sudden, transient loss of consciousness and postural tone with spontaneous recovery

Aetiology

- Generalized cerebral hypoperfusion

Clinical features

- See Fig. 6.6
- Sudden loss of consciousness
- Collapse
- Rapid recovery
- Prodrome:
    - Blurred vision
    - Sweating
    - Nausea

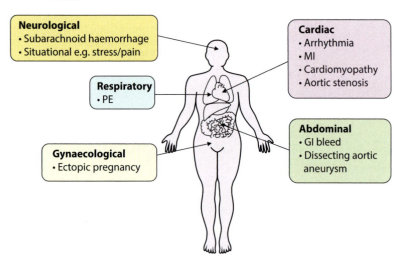

Neurological
- Subarachnoid haemorrhage
- Situational e.g. stress/pain

Respiratory
- PE

Gynaecological
- Ectopic pregnancy

Cardiac
- Arrhythmia
- MI
- Cardiomyopathy
- Aortic stenosis

Abdominal
- GI bleed
- Dissecting aortic aneurysm

Fig. 6.6 Systemic clinical features of syncope.

Investigations

- Bloods:
    - Full blood count
    - Urea and electrolytes
    - Consider arterial blood gas (check for acidosis/hypoxia)
    - Serum glucose: hypoglycaemia
    - βhCG: rule out ectopic pregnancy in women of childbearing age
- ECG: arrhythmias
- Postural blood pressure measurements: check for postural hypotension:
    - Lie flat for 5 min and check blood pressure
    - Ask patient to stand and check again after 1 and 3 min

Management

- Patient collapses in the ED/on the ward:
    - ABCDE until stable

- Patient stable/no serious cause suspected:
    - Discharge
    - Outpatient/GP follow-up
- Patient unstable/serious cause suspected:
    - Refer to relevant medical/surgical team

Syncope vs. seizure

- Differentiating syncope and seizure may be difficult (see Table 6.2)
- Detailed accounts from the patient and eyewitnesses are invaluable

Table 6.2 **Clinical features of syncope and seizures**

FEATURE	SEIZURE	SYNCOPE
Onset	Day or night Sudden	Day Gradual
Position	Any	Upright
Aura	Possible, specific aura	Dizziness Blurred vision
Colour	Normal or cyanotic	Pallor
Urinary incontinence	Common	Rare
Duration	May be prolonged	Brief
Post-ictal symptoms	May occur	Rare
Motor symptoms	May occur	Occasional jerks
Injury	Common e.g. tongue biting	Rare From falling
Automatisms	May occur e.g. absence	Do not occur

6.5 HEADACHE

Aetiology

- Common causes:
    - Tension headache
    - Migraine
- Serious/emergency causes:
    - Subarachnoid haemorrhage
    - Raised intracranial pressure
    - Meningitis
    - Temoral arteritis

- Other causes:
  - Trigeminal neuralgia
  - Cluster headache

Management

- Seek to rule out potentially serious or emergency causes of headache
- Management should be tailored to the underlying cause (see Table 6.3)

Table 6.3 **Management of headache**

DIAGNOSIS	CLINICAL FEATURES	MANAGEMENT
Tension headache	• Gradual onset over 24 h • Never during sleep • Band-like distribution	• Encourage patient to identify and modify stressors • Analgesia: NSAIDs • Discharge with GP follow-up
Migraine	• Unilateral • Throbbing • Nausea/vomiting • Photo/phonophobia • ± Preceding visual disturbance (aura)	• Analgesia • Antiemetic if nausea • Admit if serious cause cannot be ruled out • Discharge with GP follow-up, if no concern

Subarachnoid haemorrhage	• Sudden onset
	• ↑ With exertion
	• 'Worst headache', like a blow to the head
	• Usually occipital
	• Syncope
	• Nausea/vomiting
	• Meningeal signs, e.g. neck stiffness
	• Focal neurological signs, e.g. cranial nerve palsies
		• Admit
		• CT head
		  • Assess for bleeding
		  • Sensitivity ↓ with time
		• Lumbar puncture
		  • Perform if CT negative
		  • Must be >12 h after onset of symptoms to avoid false negatives
		  • Look for
		    − Xanthochromia
		    − Red blood cells
		• Prescribe analgesia plus antiemetic
		• Provide O_2
		• Urgent neurosurgery review
		  • Consider nimodipine or mannitol

(Continued)

Table 6.3 *(Continued)* **Management of headache**

DIAGNOSIS	CLINICAL FEATURES	MANAGEMENT
Raised intracranial haemorrhage	• Worst in morning • Exacerbated when supine/bending down • Vomiting • Papilloedema • Loss of retinal vein pulsation • Cranial nerve palsies	• CT scan • Urgent neurosurgery review

Meningitis	• Fever
	• Nausea/vomiting
	• Altered level of consciousness
	• Meningeal signs
	  • Neck stiffness
	  • Photophobia
	• Purpuric rash (meningococcaemia)
		• CT – if signs of raised pressure or reduced GCS
		• LP for diagnosis (see Section 18.7)
		• Treat early with
		  • Empirical antibiotics
		  • Consider steroids
		• See Section 18.7 for adults and Section 14.8 for children

Temporal arteritis (TA)	• One-sided scalp tenderness • Jaw claudication • Visual disturbances • Fever • Muscle aches • Weight loss • History of polymyalgia rheumatica	• Check ESR – elevated in TA • Give high-dose steroids immediately, if suspected • 40 mg prednisolone PO with PPI cover • Refer to neurology/rheumatology • Will need temporal artery biopsy • Urgent ophthalmology review if sight threatened
Cluster headache	• Men > women • Nocturnal headache • 'Clusters' of multiple attacks per day • Severe, unilateral pain, usually around one eye	• O_2 • Analgesia, e.g. paracetamol • Seek senior advice for consideration of ergotamine or sumatriptan treatment

(Continued)

Emergency and acute medicine

Table 6.3 *(Continued)* **Management of headache**

DIAGNOSIS	CLINICAL FEATURES	MANAGEMENT
Trigeminal neuralgia	• Unilateral, stabbing pain • Trigeminal distribution • Pain increases on stimulation of affected area e.g. combing hair	• Analgesia e.g. paracetamol • Seek senior review for consideration of carbamazepine treatment

MICRO-case

A 70-year-old woman presents to the ED with a headache. She tells you that she normally suffers with migraines, but this headache seems much worse than normal. The pain is unilateral and associated with tenderness over her right temporal area. She has been experiencing generalized muscular aches and pains and has noticed her jaw aching while chewing. She has no symptoms of visual disturbance, photophobia or nausea. There is no evidence of neck stiffness. On examination, she has a temperature of 38°C and marked tenderness over her right temple. You do not believe this is a migraine, and so choose to admit her for further tests. Blood tests show a raised ESR (103 mm/h) and a mild leukocytosis (13×10^9/L), but are otherwise normal. You suspect she has temporal arteritis. You therefore prescribe 40 mg prednisolone.

Key points:

- Steroids must be given immediately on suspicion of TA to prevent complications such as:
  - Visual loss
  - Stroke/TIA
- Always investigate a change in a patient's headache pattern.
- Always investigate a headache associated with worrying features:
  - In this case, temporal tenderness and jaw claudication
- Temporal arteritis is often associated with a raised ESR, mild fever and mild leukocytosis.
- Temporal arteritis may also present with visual disturbance, an element of headache aetiology.

6.6 GUILLAIN-BARRÉ SYNDROME

Definition
- Acute autoimmune polyneuropathy affecting the peripheral nervous system

Clinical features
- Progressive, symmetrical ascending motor weakness
- Respiratory failure secondary to diaphragmatic muscle involvement (30% will require mechanical ventilation)
- Pain, particularly in spine or limbs
- Autonomic dysfunction, including cardiac arrhythmias and labile blood pressure
- Sensory nerves usually unaffected
- Miller Fisher variant presents with a triad of ophthalmoplegia, ataxia and areflexia

Aetiology
- Autoimmune response to infective agent:
  - Campylobacter
  - CMV, EBV
  - HIV
  - Mycoplasma
  - Zoster
- Immunization
- 40% unknown

Investigations
- Bloods including FBC, clotting and inflammatory markers
- MRI to exclude other cerebral causes of symptoms
- Lumbar puncture: CSF sent for
  - Microscopy and culture to exclude infection
  - PCR for viruses
  - Elevated protein suggestive of GBS
- EMG and nerve conduction studies: may show conduction slowing acutely

Management
- Supportive care paramount including good pressure area care
- Regular forced vital capacity measurement: consider ventilation if FVC <1.5 L
- IV immunoglobulins 0.4 mg/kg daily for 5 days
- 80% of patients will make a complete recovery usually within a few months to a year

Emergency and acute medicine

7

Endocrinology and electrolyte abnormalities

7.1 DIABETIC EMERGENCIES

Definition

- Hyperglycaemic emergencies:
  - Diabetic ketoacidosis (DKA)
  - Hyperosmolar hyperglycaemic state (HHS), previously known as HONK (hyperosmolar non-ketotic diabetic state)
- Hypoglycaemia

> **MICRO-facts**
>
> Normal blood sugar: 3.5–5.5 mmol/L.

DIABETIC KETOACIDOSIS

Definition

- Triad:
  - Hyperglycaemia
  - Ketosis
  - Acidaemia

> **MICRO-facts**
>
> Although DKA is most commonly associated with type I DM, it can also occur in people with type II DM. This is more common in non-Caucasian populations, e.g. African Americans and those treated with insulin.

Epidemiology

- Type I diabetics
- May be first presentation of type I diabetes mellitus (DMI); often in young, lean individuals
- Any patient taking insulin (even type II diabetics)

Risk factors

- Poor compliance with medication
- Current illness/infection

Key features

- Thirst
- Polyuria
- Nausea and vomiting
- Abdominal pain
- Kussmaul breathing (deep, laboured, gasping hyperventilation)
- Pear drops – the smell of acetone on the breath
- Drowsiness/confusion/unconsciousness
- Dehydration:
    - ↑ HR
    - ↓ BP
    - Slow capillary refill time (≥2 s)

Investigations

- Bedside check of blood glucose
- Bloods:
    - Serum glucose: ↑
    - FBC
    - U&E
    - Venous bicarbonate: ≤16 = acidosis
    - HbA1c – assess overall glycaemic control
- Urine dipstick: ↑ glucose and ketones
- Urinary pregacy test in women of childbearing age
- ECG: if >30 years of age, rule out MI
- Consider the following in suspected infection:
    - CXR
    - Blood cultures: MC&S
    - Urine: MC&S

> ### MICRO-facts
>
> For immediate results, venous HCO_3^- and K^+ may be analyzed using a blood gas machine.

Management

- Basic:
    - ABC
    - Commence IV fluids urgently

- Ensure passing urine
- Consider giving antibiotics if clinical evidence of infection
- Prophylactic LMWH subcutaneously once daily
- IV fluids, patients on presentation can be 4–6 L in deficit
- Insulin, potassium: see Fig. 7.1

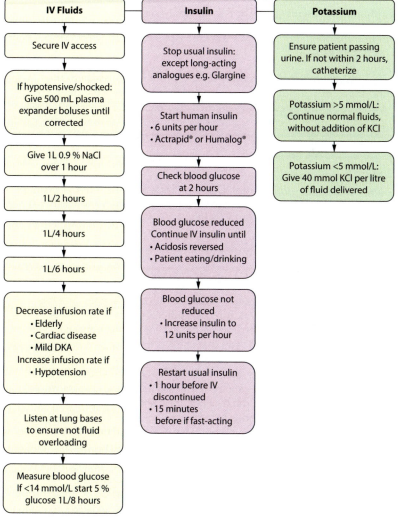

Fig. 7.1 Management of DKA.

Emergency and acute medicine

Monitoring

- Check the following, initially 2-hourly with a venous gas:
  - Venous HCO_3^-
  - Serum glucose
  - Serum K^+
- Check U&E at 2, 4 and 8 h
- Monitor vital signs (BP, HR, RR and SpO_2) regularly

MICRO-facts

Hyperglycaemia increases the viscosity of the blood, so there is an increased risk of clot formation. LMWH is given to prevent deep vein thrombosis. This is especially important in unconscious and immobile patients.

MICRO-reference

DKA Guidelines – Joint British Diabetes Societies Inpatient Care Group: Management of Diabetic Ketoacidosis in Adults. http://www.diabetes.org.uk/Documents/About%20Us/What%20we%20say/Management-of-DKA-241013.pdf

---

MICRO-case

A 14-year-old girl presents to the ED with abdominal pain. She has been vomiting this morning, but does not have diarrhoea. She is breathing rapidly and interrupts you to ask for a drink because she is very thirsty. Her father tells you that she has lost a lot of weight recently. On examination, you note that she is extremely slim. She is tachycardic and hypotensive. Her skin feels cool and dry and her abdomen is soft. You smell her breath, but cannot detect any abnormal odours. You check her blood glucose, dipstick her urine and take a venous blood sample. Her BM is 16, venous bicarbonate is 10 mmol/L and her urine is positive for ketones. When you get back, you notice that her breathing has become very deep and laboured. You diagnose her as having DKA.

- 25% of those diagnosed with type I diabetes first present in DKA.
- Rapid weight loss is a key feature of new type I diabetes.
- Ketone bodies in the blood create a metabolic acidosis. Respiratory compensation occurs as hyperventilation – rapid, shallow breathing. This is an early sign and is succeeded by deeper, more laboured 'Kussmaul breathing'.

continued...

continued...

- Abdominal pain is often associated with DKA and can sometimes be confused for an acute surgical abdomen. Glucose must always be tested on admission to rule this out.
- Blood glucose metre monitoring is not completely accurate, so serum glucose levels must be used to confirm results.
  - The smell of acetone on the breath is definitive for DKA, but its absence cannot rule out the condition.
  - Urinary ketones must be investigated with a urine dip.

HYPEROSMOLAR HYPERGLYCAEMIC STATE (HHS)

Definition

- Hyperglycaemia: serum glucose usually ≥50 mmol/L
- Hyperosmolality: usually ≥330 mOsm/kg
- Venous bicarbonate: ≥20 mmol/L

MICRO-print
Osmolality can be obtained from the lab as a part of your routine investigation of HHS, but it can be calculated on the ward using the following equation:

$$2 [Na^+ + K^+] + BG$$

Risk factors

- Type II diabetes
- ↑ Age
- Obesity
- Newly diagnosed diabetes
- Recent infection/illness

Clinical features

- Thirst
- Polyuria
- Nausea
- Disorientation
- Dehydration:
  - ↑ HR
  - ↓ BP
  - Slow capillary refill time (≥2 s)

Emergency and acute medicine

- Drowsiness
- Focal neurological deficits
- ↓ Level of consciousness

Investigations and management

- Follow protocol for DKA
- Monitor sodium levels, which rise as glucose level falls
  - If ≥155 mmol/L, consider switching fluids to 0.45% NaCl
- Closely monitor fluids as depletion may be severe

DKA vs. HHS

- See Table 7.1

Table 7.1 **Differentiating features between DKA and HHS**

DIFFERENTIATING FEATURES	DKA	HHS
Type	Type I DM (rarely II)	Type II DM
Demographics	Young Lean	Older Any body habitus
Onset	Rapid (≤24 h)	Gradual (days–weeks)
Blood glucose	Usually 11–17 mmol/L, but may be greater	≥50 mmol/L
Volume depletion	Present	Severe
Abdominal pain	Common	Rare
Confusion	Rare	Common
Focal neurology	No	Sometimes

HYPOGLYCAEMIA

Definition

- Blood glucose <4 mmol/L associated with clinical symptoms, which resolve on the correction of blood glucose levels

> ## MICRO-facts
> - Hypoglycaemia can mimic any neurological deficit.
> - Check glucose in all patients with altered consciousness or focal neurology.

Risk factors

- Type I and type II diabetes
- Insulin therapy
- Elderly (falls)
- Alcohol/drug abuse
- Fasting, e.g. religious
- Exercise
- Shift workers
- Exogenous insulin e.g. insulin secreting tumour
- Ingestion of oral hypoglycaemics

Clinical features

- Autonomic and neuroglycopaenic symptoms are shown in Table 7.2

Table 7.2 **Clinical features of hypoglycaemic states**

AUTONOMIC	NEUROGLYCOPAENIC
Early Serum glucose 3.3–3.6 mmol/L	Late Serum glucose ≤2.6 mmol/L
Sweating	Tiredness
Anxiety	Poor coordination
Nausea	Visual disturbances
Palpitations	Drowsiness
Hunger	Altered behaviour
Paraesthesia	Confusion
	Ataxia
	Focal neuropathy
	Seizures
	Coma

MICRO-facts

Never omit next dose of insulin in **type I diabetics,** as this may precipitate DKA. The next dose may be omitted in **type II diabetics** if **severe** hypoglycaemia (≤3 mmol/L).

Emergency and acute medicine

7.2 HYPOADRENAL (ADDISONIAN) CRISIS

Definition
- Adrenal insufficiency resulting in deficiency of glucocorticoid

Aetiology
- Sudden cessation of chronic steroid treatment
- Addison's disease exacerbated by infection, injury or stress which increase steroid requirement

Clinical features
- Shock:
  - ↑HR
  - ↓BP
  - ↓ Urine output
- Hypoglycaemia:
  - Confusion
  - ↓ Level of consciousness
- Hyperpigmentation: Secondary to Addison's disease

Investigations
- Serum potassium: ↑
- Serum calcium: ↑
- Serum uric acid: ↑
- Serum sodium: ↓

Management
- ABC
- IV fluids:
  - 1 L of normal saline stat
  - Or plasma expander if very hypotensive
  - Further litres of normal saline according to response
- Hydrocortisone:
  - 100 mg IV initially
  - At least 50 mg IM every 6 h until better (IM doses prevent a rapid drop-off in steroid levels)
- Glucose IV (if hypoglycaemic)
- Investigate and treat precipitant cause e.g. infection

7.3 THYROTOXIC CRISIS

Epidemiology
- Usually known hyperthyroidism
- May be initial presentation of hyperthyroidism

Aetiology
- Infection
- Stress
- Surgery
- Iatrogenic:
    - Radioactive iodine therapy
    - Inappropriate cessation of anti-thyroid therapy

Clinical features
- Tachycardia, atrial fibrillation
- Restlessness
- Hyperpyrexia
- Confusion
- Pulmonary oedema (rare)

Investigations
- FBC: raised WCC suggesting infection
- U&Es
- Glucose
- TFTs: raised thyroxine or triiodothyronine
- Cultures
- ECG: AF/tachycardia
- CXR: features of heart failure may be present

Management
- ABC
- IV propanolol, carbimazole, iodine, dexamethasone
- Treat precipitating factors

7.4 ELECTROLYTE ABNORMALITIES

HYPONATRAEMIA

Definition
- Na^+ <135 mmol/L
- Severe (Na^+ <120 mmol/L)

> ## MICRO-facts
>
> Normal range of Na$^+$ = 135–145 mmol/L

> **MICRO-print**
>
> Pseudohyponatraemia occurs when there are falsely low levels of Na$^+$ due to:
> - Very high circulating levels of lipids or proteins
> - Intracellular water pushed into the extracellular space

Aetiology

- See Fig. 7.2

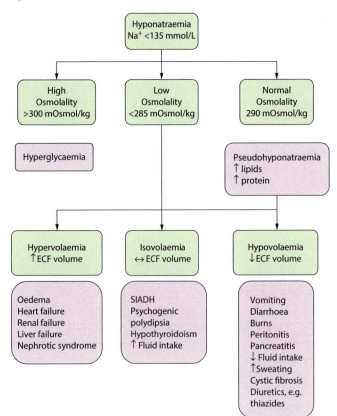

Fig. 7.2 Aetiology of hyponatraemia.

- Na⁺ loss through urine.
- Increased fluid in the blood:
  - Drinking excess water
  - Water retention
  - Decreased urine production
  - Osmotically active agents e.g. glucose
- ECF = extracellular fluid volume; determined by sodium concentration and relies upon tight physiological control
- In hyponatraemia there is a decreased Na⁺:water ratio in the ECF

MICRO-facts

Increased serum osmolality occurs due to:
- Decreased water in the blood
- Increased solutes in the blood

Decreased serum osmolality occurs due to:
- Increased fluid levels

Clinical features

- See Fig. 7.3

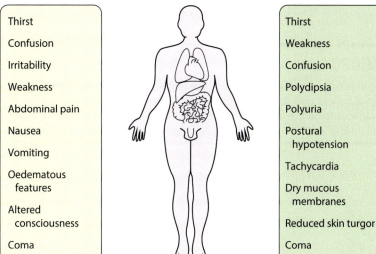

HYPONANATRAEMIA

| Thirst |
| Confusion |
| Irritability |
| Weakness |
| Abdominal pain |
| Nausea |
| Vomiting |
| Oedematous features |
| Altered consciousness |
| Coma |

HYPERNATRAEMIA

| Thirst |
| Weakness |
| Confusion |
| Polydipsia |
| Polyuria |
| Postural hypotension |
| Tachycardia |
| Dry mucous membranes |
| Reduced skin turgor |
| Coma |

Fig. 7.3 Clinical features of hyponatraemia and hypernatraemia.

Investigations

- Fluid charts
- Serum sodium
- U&Es
- Serum glucose
- Plasma osmolality
  - Normal: consider pseudohyponatraemia
  - Low: further investigation
  - High: most likely to be hyperglycaemia
- Urine sodium: >20 mmol/L likely inappropriate sodium excretion
- CXR: looking for lung cancer in SIADH
- Review medications: anti-epileptics, antidepressants, diuretics and PPIs can all cause hyponatraemia

Management

- If mild, no treatment is needed. Correct the underlying cause.
- If symptomatic or very high levels:
  - ABC
- If very unwell, consider management in critical care:
  - Severe CNS symptoms: hypertonic (1.8%, 3%) saline – *do not* give without discussion with seniors
  - Hypovolaemic: replace fluid loss with 0.9% saline and stop diuretics
  - Euvolaemic: fluid restriction to 1500 mL/24 h until Na^+ corrects
  - Hypervolaemic: furosemide and ACE inhibitors
  - SIADH can be managed long term with fluid restriction, demeclocyline or vasopressin receptor antagonists

---

MICRO-facts

Correcting hyponatraemia too quickly can lead to central pontine myelinolysis and cerebral oedema due to large shifts of intracellular water outside the brainstem and pons. Aim to correct at no more than 10 mmol/L per 24 h.

HYPERNATRAEMIA

Definition

- Na^+ >145 mmol/L

Aetiology

- See Table 7.3

Table 7.3 **Aetiology of hypernatraemia**

HYPOVOLAEMIA	NORMOVOLAEMIA	HYPERVOLAEMIA
Burns	Diabetes insipidus	Use of hypertonic saline
Excessive sweating	Pituitary: failure of ADH secretion	Tube feeding

GI losses
   Diarrhoea
   Vomiting
   Fistulae
	Nephrogenic: failure of ADH response	IV antibiotics with sodium

Osmotic diuresis e.g. DKA	Impaired thirst (e.g. dementia)	Hypertonic dialysis
Diuretics	Fever	Hyperaldosteronism
Post-obstruction	Hyperventilation	Excess salt ingestion
Acute/chronic renal failure	Mechanical ventilation	
HHS coma		

Clinical features

- See Fig. 7.3

Investigations

- Fluid charts: measure fluid intake and losses
- Serum sodium level
- Serum glucose level: diabetes mellitus
- Urine and serum osmolality: diabetes insipidus
- Imaging: head CT or MRI if *severe* for head injury or central diabetes insipidus suspected

Management

- ABC
- Fluid volume resuscitation: usually normal saline is appropriate in dehydrated patients
- Decrease urine volume: salt restriction, thiazide diuretics
- Hypovolaemic: 0.9% saline slowly unless the patient is in severe shock (avoid rapid correction!)
- Normovolaemic: oral fluids
- Insert urinary cathether: assess urine output
- Haemodialysis: if patient is in renal failure

It is important to recheck electrolytes frequently during fluid correction!

> **MICRO-case**
>
> A 29-year-old male is brought into the ED by the paramedics with severe head trauma and multiple lacerations from an RTA. He was previously well with no significant past medical history, and he is not taking any regular medication.
>
> A head CT reveals some intracranial haemorrhage and cerebral oedema. During his inpatient stay, his mental state progressively deteriorated.
>
> He is normovolaemic and normotensive.
>
> ABG is performed and blood gases on room air show: pH 7.39, pCO_2 5.3, pO_2 10.5.
>
> IV access is obtained and blood tests are performed which were as follows: serum Na^+ 110, K^+ 4.1, urea 3.3, Cr 100, glucose 5.2, plasma osmolality 260. The low plasma osmolality is investigated further with a urine test sent to biochemistry, which revealed urine sodium 45 mmol/L and urine osmolality 300 mOsm/kg. Thyroid function and adrenal function are normal. The tests suggest hyponatraemia due to SIADH.
>
> The patient is transferred to ITU and started on hypertonic saline aiming to correct his hyponatraemia no faster than 10 mmol/L in 24 h.
>
> **Learning points:**
> - A common cause of hyponatraemia is syndrome of inappropriate ADH or SIADH that can occur after severe head injury.
> - Hyponatraemia occurs by abnormally high secretion of ADH.
> - In SIADH, there is low plasma sodium, low plasma osmolality and high urine osmolality (concentrated urine) and high urine sodium.
> - First-line treatment of hyponatraemia without significant neurological impairment is fluid restriction to 1.5 L/24 h.
> - Important to check U&Es, glucose and blood gases in an unconscious patient to exclude reversible causes.
> - Assess volume status and monitor with fluid charts in hyponatraemia.
> - Important to assess renal, adrenal and thyroid function.

CALCIUM (CA^{2+}) DISTURBANCES

- Calcium is mainly bound to albumin or exists in bone
- Unbound ionized Ca^{2+} is active
- Calcium is important in:
  - Bone formation
  - Nerve depolarization
  - Skeletal and cardiac muscle contraction
- Ca is regulated primarily by parathyroid hormone (PTH), vitamin D and calcitonin

- Low-serum Ca^{2+} stimulates PTH release, which in turn raises serum Ca^{2+} by increasing bone resorption, renal absorption and activates vitamin D to increase intestinal and bone absorption
- Raised Ca^{2+} stops PTH release and calcitonin is released, which increases resorption of calcium from bone and excretion by the kidneys
- Ca^{2+} disturbances arise when there is a disturbance in any of the regulatory hormones or their secretory organs

HYPOCALCAEMIA

Definition

- Ca^{2+} <2.10 mmol/L

MICRO-facts

Normal Ca^{2+} range = 2.10–2.60 mmol/L

Aetiology

- See Table 7.4

Table 7.4 **Aetiology of hypocalcaemia**

CAUSES OF HYPOCALCAEMIA	AETIOLOGY
Hyperphosphataemia	• Chronic renal failure

Hypoparathyroidism	• Neck surgery
	  • Thyroidectomy
	  • Parathyroidectomy
	• Irradiation
	• Idiopathic

Vitamin D deficiency	• Osteomalacia/rickets • Malabsorption • Sepsis
Hypomagnesaemia	• Diarrhoea
Medication	• Calcitonin • Bisphosphonates • Anticonvulsants
Rhabdomyolysis	• Prolonged seizures or found on floor
Acute pancreatitis	e.g. Following ERCP

Emergency and acute medicine

Clinical features

● See Fig. 7.4

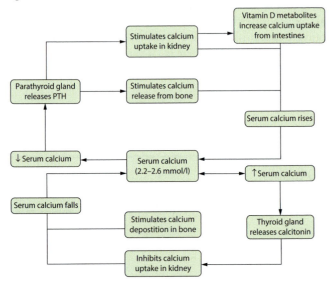

Fig. 7.4 Physiology of calcium regulation.

Investigations

● ECG:
  ○ Prolonged QT interval
  ○ Sinus bradycardia
  ○ Complete heart block
  ○ T wave inversion
  ○ Arrythmias
● Blood tests:
  ○ Total serum calcium: <2.5 mmol/L
  ○ Ionized calcium: <2.0 mEq/L
  ○ U&Es: renal failure
  ○ Serum amylase: acute pancreatitis
  ○ Creatinine kinase: rhabdomyloysis
  ○ Serum magnesium and phosphate (low Mg^{2+} causes low Ca^{2+})
  ○ Serum albumin: the amount of biologically inactive calcium which is bound
  ○ Serum PTH levels
  ○ Vitamin D serum levels (may be low)
● X-ray:
  ○ Fracture
  ○ Radiolucency

Management

- The underlying cause should be investigated and treated accordingly

> **MICRO-print**
> Patients on digoxin have increased cardiac sensitivity to changes in calcium levels; therefore treatment with IV calcium should be approached with more caution and continuous ECG monitoring to avoid digoxin toxicity.

- Symptomatic or Ca^{2+} <1.90 mmol/L:
  - ECG monitoring
  - IV calcium gluconate: 10 mL of 10% solution over 10 min
  - Regular calcium level monitoring
  - Oral vitamin D
  - Correction of other electrolytes: in hypomagnesaemia, hypocalcaemia will not resolve
- Asymptomatic: oral calcium therapy with vitamin D analogue (calcitriol) at home

Hypercalcaemia
Definition

- Ca^{2+} >2.60 mmol/L

Aetiology

- See Table 7.5

Table 7.5 **Aetiology of hypercalcaemia**

CAUSES	AETIOLOGY
Primary hyperparathyroidism	Parathyroid adenoma Parathyroid hyperplasia Parathyroid carcinoma Multiple endocrine neoplasia 1 and 2A
Malignancy	Bone metastases Myeloma PTH secreting tumours – breast and lung cancers (squamous cell)
Excess vitamin D intake	Excess supplementation
Hyperthyroidism	Thyrotoxicosis
Drugs	Thiazide diuretics Lithium Vitamin A
Granulomatous disorders	TB Sarcoidosis

Clinical features

- Mostly related to the effect on neuromuscular function; see Fig. 7.5

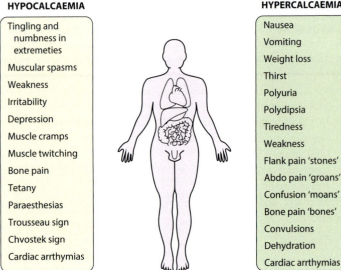

HYPOCALCAEMIA

- Tingling and numbness in extremeties
- Muscular spasms
- Weakness
- Irritability
- Depression
- Muscle cramps
- Muscle twitching
- Bone pain
- Tetany
- Paraesthesias
- Trousseau sign
- Chvostek sign
- Cardiac arrthymias

HYPERCALCAEMIA

- Nausea
- Vomiting
- Weight loss
- Thirst
- Polyuria
- Polydipsia
- Tiredness
- Weakness
- Flank pain 'stones'
- Abdo pain 'groans'
- Confusion 'moans'
- Bone pain 'bones'
- Convulsions
- Dehydration
- Cardiac arrthymias

Fig. 7.5 Clinical features of hypo- and hypercalcaemia.

Investigations

- ECG:
  - Short QT interval
  - Prolonged PR interval
  - Broad QRS complex and T wave inversion (severe)
  - Sinus bradycardia
  - Cardiac arrythmias
- Blood:
  - U&Es: serum calcium, phosphate, ALP
  - TFTs (low calcium in hypothyroidism) (see Table 7.6)
  - Serum PTH
  - ESR (significantly raised in myeloma)
  - PTHrP assay
  - Serum albumin: bound to calcium
- Serum and urine electrophoresis: myeloma (Bence-Jones protein)
- 24 h urine collection: calcium/creatinine clearance
- Imaging:
  - CXR: pathological fractures, bone metastases
  - Bone density scan
  - USS/CT: renal stones

Table 7.6 **Biochemistry results typically found in some conditions related to altering calcium levels**

CONDITION	CA^{2+}	PO_4^{3-}	PTH	ALP
Bone metastases	↑	↔	↓	↑
Primary hyperparathyroidism	↑	↓	↑	↑
Hypoparathyroidism	↓	↑	↓	↔
Osteomalacia/rickets	↓	↓	↑	↑
Vitamin D deficiency/malabsorption	↓	↓	↑	↑

MICRO-print

Serum calcium exists as ionized free calcium which is biologically active or bound to albumin; therefore serum calcium concentration needs to be interpreted in relation to serum albumin (commonly referred to as adjusted Ca^{2+}).

For every 1 g/L ± the reference value of albumin (40 g/L), calcium is corrected by ↑ or ↓ by 0.02 mmol/L.

Management

- In acute hypercalcaemia, it is important to control/reduce calcium level and ensure adequate hydration, then treat the underlying cause
- Symptomatic: particularly dehydrated and altered consciousness
  - IV fluids: 1–2 L of normal 0.9% saline: increase urinary excretion of calcium
  - IV bisphosphonates: palmidronate in 0.9% saline, reduce bone turnover
  - IV/oral furosemide: increase urinary excretion of calcium and inhibit tubular reabsorption. Only give after dehydration is corrected!
  - ECG monitoring
  - Prednisolone: hypercalcaemia secondary to granulomatous diseases
  - Dialysis: hypercalcaemia secondary to renal failure
  - Investigate cause

POTASSIUM DISTURBANCES

- Potassium (K^+) is the main intracellular cation
- It determines cellular membrane resting potential
- This controls nervous and muscle function
- Serum K^+ levels are controlled by:
  - Renal excretion
  - Extrarenal losses
  - Balance between intracellular and extracellular fluids under the control of the hormone aldosterone

Emergency and acute medicine

Hypokalaemia
Definition

- K⁺ <3.5 mEq/L
- Severe (K⁺ <2.5 mEql/L) or ECG changes

> **MICRO-facts**
>
> Normal K⁺ range = 3.5–5.5 mEq/L

Aetiology

- Vomiting and/or diarrhoea
- Hypovolaemia
- Alkalosis
- Thiazide and loop diuretics
- Laxative
- Bulimia nervosa
- Steroids
- Conn syndrome

Clinical features

- See Fig. 7.6

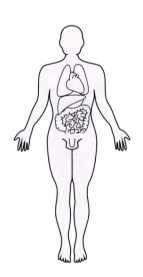

HYPOKALAEMIA

Generalized weakness
Cramps
Chest pain
Palpitations
Dizziness
Paraesthesia
Tetany
Thirst
Polyuria
Psychosis
Hypotension
Hypoventilation
Reduced muscle strength
Reduced tendon reflexes
Oedema
Ileus
Sudden death

HYPERKALAEMIA

Weakness
Fatigue
Shortness of breath
Chest pain
Palpitations
Nausea
Vomiting
Cramps
Paraesthesias
Paralysis
Tetany
Bradycardia
Tachnypnoea
Cardiac arrthymias
Sudden death

Fig. 7.6 Clinical features of hypokalaemia and hyperkalaemia.

Investigations
- Blood tests:
  - U&Es: potassium level (low), magnesium (if low, then needs to be treated; otherwise hypokalaemia resistant to treatment)
  - ABG: if unwell (may show metabolic alkalosis)
- ECG: monitor cardiac function and assess for digoxin toxicity
  - Prolonged PR interval, ST depression, inverted or small T waves

Management
- ABC
- 15 L/min oxygen
- Continuous ECG monitoring, BP, pulse oximetry
- Replace K^+: 20–40 mml IV KCl 1 L in 0.9% saline at a rate not faster than over 60 min and oral K^+
- Mild: oral K^+: e.g. Sando-K®
- Monitor U&Es

Hyperkalaemia
Definition
- K^+ >5.5 mEq/L

Aetiology
- Common and important:
  - Acute renal failure
  - ACE inhibitors
  - K^+ sparing diuretics: Amiloride, spironolactone
- See Table 7.7

Clinical features
- See Fig. 7.6

Investigations
- Blood tests:
  - U&E: potassium level
    - Mild (K^+ >5.3 mmol/L)
    - Moderate (K^+ 6.1–6.9 mmol/L)
    - Severe (K^+ >7 mmol/L)
  - Repeat U&E urgently: if the first sample was haemolyzed and assess renal function
  - Serum calcium
  - Glucose
  - Venous gas: metabolic acidosis and check K^+ level

Emergency and acute medicine

Table 7.7 **Aetiology of hyperkalaemia**

CAUSE	AETIOLOGY
Pseudohyperkalaemia	Haemolyzed sample Marked leucocytosis Thrombocytosis
Increased K⁺ load	Blood transfusions Rhabdomyolysis: crush injuries Burns Potassium supplements
Decreased renal excretion	Acute or chronic renal failure Hypoaldosteronism – Addisonian crisis Renal tubular acidosis ACE inhibitors NSAIDs K⁺ sparing diuretics: spironolactone
Transcellular shift of K⁺ out of cells	Metabolic acidosis: DKA Medications: beta-blockers, digoxin toxicity

- ECG (see Fig. 7.7):
  - Tented T waves
  - Broad QRS complex
  - Prolonged PR interval
  - Absent P waves
  - VF/VT
- Urinalysis: if signs of renal failure

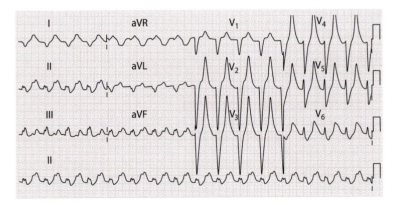

Fig. 7.7 ECG changes in hyperkalaemia.

MICRO-facts

Hyperkalaemia is life-threatening.
Urgent management if K$^+$ >6 mEq/L or there are ECG changes:

- Tented T waves
- Prolonged PR interval
- Absent P waves
- Broad QRS complex

MICRO-print
Ca^{2+} antagonizes the effects of extracellular K$^+$ on cardiac function.

Management

- ABC
- 15 L/min oxygen
- IV access
- Continuous ECG monitoring
- 10 mL of 10% calcium gluconate IV over 10 min: protects myocardium
- 10 units of short-acting insulin in 50 mL of 50% dextrose IV over 20 min: increase cellular uptake of K$^+$
- 10 mg nebulized salbutamol: increases cellular uptake of K$^+$
- Correct fluid volume/acidosis: IV fluids
- Correct underlying cause
- If K$^+$ does not respond to medical treatment, then refer to nephrologists for potential dialysis
- Oral or rectal calcium resonium to reduce the total body potassium; all of the above measures just move the K$^+$ from the blood and it will return
- Mild hyperkalaemia: IV fluid: treat associated hypovolaemia/fluid loss/acidosis

MICRO-facts

Hyperkalaemia in cardiac arrest:

- Advanced life support
- 10 mL of 10% IV calcium chloride as rapid bolus
- 50 mmol sodium bicarbonate rapid IV (in severe metabolic acidosis/renal failure)
- 10 units of short-acting insulin plus 50 mL of 50% glucose rapid IV

Emergency and acute medicine

MICRO-case

A 55-year-old male with diabetes mellitus, essential hypertension and gout presents to the ED with acute abdominal pain, palpitations and generalized weakness. He has normal renal function. His K^+ is phoned through from the lab at 7.9 mmol/L, and his ECG reveals bradycardia, wide QRS complexes, first degree heart block and peaked T waves. Treatment is commenced with IV fluids, calcium gluconate, insulin and dextrose infusion. The patient is admitted to the ward with cardiac montoring, and repeat bloods are sent. The hyperkalaemia resolves to 5.3 mmol/L and urea and creatinine are normal; therefore the patient does not require dialysis therapy.

The ECG also reverts to sinus rhythm with a rate of 86/min and normal T waves.

Learning points:

- Hyperkalaemia is a potentially life-threatening condition with non-specific clinical features.
- Hyperkalaemia can lead to sudden death from cardiac arrythmias; therefore an urgent ECG is required for all patients with suspected hyperkalaemia.
- Initial management is assessment of ABC and ECG monitoring to assess cardiac status.
- If there are ECG signs, treatment is IV access, fluids, calcium gluconate IV, IV insulin and 50 mL of 50% dextrose infusion, and nebulized salbutamol.
- Dialysis is not always necessary for severe hyperkalaemia and may only be needed in patients with acute or chronic renal failure or with life-threatening hyperkalaemia unresponsive to first-line treatments.

8 Renal emergencies

8.1 ACUTE KIDNEY INJURY

Definitions
- Acute kidney injury (AKI): deterioration in renal function and glomerular filtration rate over hours to days
- Acute-on-chronic kidney failure: exacerbation of pre-existing renal failure often due to intercurrent illness, obstruction and infection

Features
- Raised urea and creatinine
- ± Oliguria/anuria
- Symptoms and signs of cause

> **MICRO-facts**
>
> Oliguria: Urine output <0.5 mL/kg/h or <500 mL/day
> Anuria: Urine output <50 mL/day

Epidemiology and risk factors
- Elderly
- Diabetes mellitus
- Hypertension
- Vascular disease
- Pre-existing renal disease
- Critically ill patient

Consequences of abnormal renal function
- See table 8.1

Table 8.1 **Consequences of abnormal renal function**

NORMAL RENAL FUNCTION	CONSEQUENCE OF RENAL FAILURE
Maintain fluid balance	• Water overload or depletion • Effect on blood pressure
Electrolyte balance	• Electrolyte disturbances, e.g. $\uparrow K^+/\uparrow Na$
Acid base balance	• Metabolic acidosis
Removal of toxins	• Reduced drug and nitrogenous waste excretion
Endocrine	• Failure of erythropoietin production and vitamin D hydroxylation

Clinical features

● See Fig. 8.1

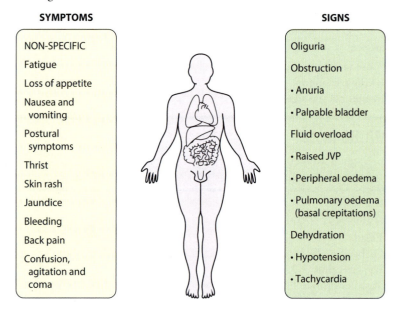

SYMPTOMS

NON-SPECIFIC

Fatigue

Loss of appetite

Nausea and vomiting

Postural symptoms

Thrist

Skin rash

Jaundice

Bleeding

Back pain

Confusion, agitation and coma

SIGNS

Oliguria

Obstruction

• Anuria

• Palpable bladder

Fluid overload

• Raised JVP

• Peripheral oedema

• Pulmonary oedema (basal crepitations)

Dehydration

• Hypotension

• Tachycardia

Fig. 8.1 Clinical features of renal failure.

MICRO-facts

Chronic renal failure may be asymptomatic and present as an incidental finding on blood results.

Aetiology

- See Table 8.2
- Hypovolaemia
- Glomerulonephritis
- Sepsis
- Drugs
- Obstruction

Table 8.2 **Aetiology of renal failure divided by anatomical location**

PRE-RENAL	RENAL	POST-RENAL
<ul><li>Hypovolaemia:<ul><li>Dehydration</li><li>Haemorrhage</li><li>Sepsis</li></ul></li><li>Hypoperfusion:<ul><li>Renal artery stenosis</li><li>NSAIDs</li></ul></li><li>Hypotension/shock</li><li>Oedema:<ul><li>Cardiac failure</li><li>Nephrotic syndrome</li></ul></li></ul>	<ul><li>Glomerulonephritis</li><li>Tubular:<ul><li>Acute tubular necrosis</li><li>Toxins/drugs</li><li>Radio-contrast media</li></ul></li><li>Interstitial nephritis:<ul><li>Drug induced</li><li>Infective</li><li>Granulomatous TB</li><li>Sarcoidosis</li></ul></li><li>Vascular:<ul><li>Vasculitis</li><li>DIC</li><li>TTP</li><li>Renal artery thrombosis</li></ul></li></ul>	<ul><li>Prostatic hypertrophy</li><li>Ureteric stones</li><li>Ureteric trauma</li></ul>

Investigations

- Urinalysis:
  - Dipstick:
    - Haematuria: glomerulonephritis or calculi
    - Proteinuria
    - Leucocytes
    - Nitrites
    - Glucose
  - Microscopy:
    - RBCs
    - WBCs
    - Red cell casts (glomerulonephritis)
    - Crystals
    - Culture and sensitivity
    - Bence-Jones protein

- Bloods:
  - U&E: ↑ urea and creatinine, maybe ↑ K+
  - Serum bicarbonate: ↓ in metabolic acidosis
  - ESR and protein electrophoresis (myeloma)
  - CRP
  - LFTs (hepatorenal syndrome)
  - Blood cultures (if suspected sepsis)
  - Immunology – ANCA, complement, immunoglobulins, ANA, double-stranded DNA, anti-GBM (if glomerulonephritis suspected)
  - eGFR – assess severity of renal impairment (more accurate measure of chronic renal impairment than urea and creatinine). See Table 8.3
  - ABG: metabolic acidosis, check K+
- Radiology:
  - Renal USS
  - X-ray KUB – to look for stones
  - CT-KUB is gold standard test to look for stones
- ECG (signs of hyperkalaemia)

Table 8.3 **Calculated eGFR and the corresponding stage of CKD**

EGFR (ML/MIN/1.73 M^2)	CKD STAGE	DESCRIPTION
>90	0–1	Normal kidneys unless other evidence present
60–89	2	Mild impairment
45–59 30–44	3A 3B	Moderate impairment
15–29	4	Severe impairment
<15	5	End-stage disease requiring dialysis or transplant

Management

- See Fig. 8.2

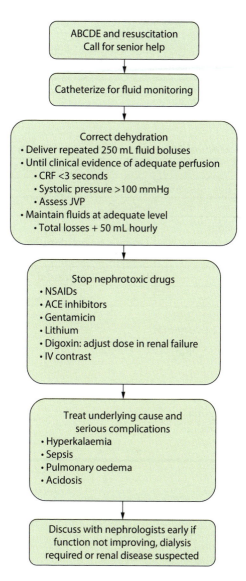

Fig. 8.2 Management of acute renal failure.

MICRO-facts

Management of hyperkalaemia
- 10 mL of 10% calcium gluconate over 2 min
- 50 mL of IV dextrose (50%) with 10 units of Actrapid insulin
- 5 mg nebulized salbutamol

Indications for haemodialysis/haemofiltration

- See Table 8.4

Table 8.4 Complications of ARF and their indications for dialysis

COMPLICATION	INDICATION FOR DIALYSIS
Severe persisting hyperkalaemia	>6 mmol/L
Acidosis	pH <7.2
Symptomatic uraemia	Urea >50 Uraemic encephalopathy: low GCS/seizures Uraemic pericarditis: chest pain
Pulmonary oedema	If diuresis unsuccessful
Coma	

Indicators of a poor prognosis

- Age >50
- Sepsis
- Burns
- Rising urea (>16)
- Persisting oliguria
- Multi-organ failure
- Jaundice

MICRO-facts

Life threatening consequences of AKI, which are important to remember and treat:
- Hyperkalaemia
- Pulmonary oedema
- Metabolic acidosis

MICRO-reference

NICE Guidelines for Acute Kidney Injury, http://publications.nice.org.uk/acute-kidney-injury-cg169

MICRO-case

A 65-year-old male is referred to hospital by his GP after routine blood results reveal his urea to be 65 mmol/L, creatinine 650 μmol/L and K+ 7.1 mmol/L. He has been feeling increasingly tired and nauseated over the last week and had some episodes of diarrhoea and vomiting. The patient has type II diabetes and hypertension.

On admission, the patient's initial observations reveal a pulse rate of 101 bpm, blood pressure 138/78 mmHg, respiratory rate of 16 breaths/min and oxygen saturation of 99% on air. On clinical examination, there are no respiratory or cardiac abnormalities. IV access is obtained and further blood is taken.

A venous gas is performed which confirms severe hyperkalaemia, and an ECG shows some peaked T waves and broad complexes. He is attached to a cardiac monitor and treated with calcium gluconate and an IV insulin and glucose infusion.

The patient appears clinically dehydrated and is therefore given IV fluid resuscitation of 250 mL 0.9% saline over 15 min. He has not passed any urine since arrival; therefore a urinary catheter is inserted which drains 75 mL concentrated urine. A further 500 mL of 0.9% saline is given over 30 min.

His repeat potassium level after the above treatment is 5.9 and his ECG changes have resolved on repeat trace. His antihypertensive medication is withheld and insulin is continued for his diabetes and potassium level. IV fluids are continued with regular fluid assessments to titrate rate.

Key points:
- A history of diabetes and hypertension could result in renal vascular disease causing chronic renal impairment.
- Diarrhoea and vomiting cause excess fluid losses, and combined poor oral fluid intake could result in hypovolaemia leading to acute-on-chronic renal failure.
- Medications such as ACE inhibitors could contribute to poor renal perfusion in the context of hypovolaemia.
- Initial management should be resuscitative care (ABC).
- An ECG is essential in symptomatic and asymptomatic patients as hyperkalaemia is a serious complication of acute renal failure.
- If fluid resuscitation is required, review patient's fluid status regularly to monitor any fluid overload which can manifest as pulmonary oedema.
- Once the complications have been managed and the patient is more stable, it is important to identify the underlying cause for the deterioration in renal function.

Emergency and acute medicine

8.2 URINARY TRACT INFECTION (UTI)

Pathophysiology
- See Fig. 8.3
- Lower UTI (cystitis): bladder infection via urethra
- Upper UTI (pyelonephritis): proximal infection via ureters

Microbiology
- Most common organisms:
  - *E. coli* (90%)
  - *Proteus* spp., *Klebsiella* spp., *Staphylococcus* spp.
  - *Pseudomonas aeruginosa*: indwelling catheter

Risk factors
- Diabetes mellitus
- Pregnancy
- Obstruction: Impaired voiding
- Genitourinary malformation
- Sexual intercourse
- Bladder calculi
- Neurogenic bladder

Clinical features
- More common in women, due to a shorter urethra
- In males, UTIs are more common at extremes of age

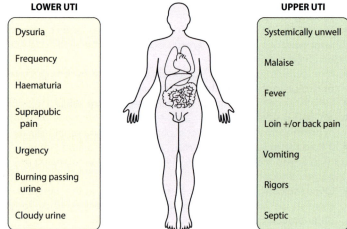

LOWER UTI	UPPER UTI
Dysuria	Systemically unwell
Frequency	Malaise
Haematuria	Fever
Suprapubic pain	Loin +/or back pain
Urgency	Vomiting
Burning passing urine	Rigors
Cloudy urine	Septic

Fig. 8.3 Comparison of lower UTI and pyelonephritis.

Emergency and acute medicine

> **MICRO-facts**
>
> It is important to exclude a UTI in elderly patients who present with confusion.

Investigations

- Lower and upper UTI:
  - Urinalysis:
    - Urine dip: nitrites, leucocytes, blood, protein.
    - MC&S: white blood cells, red blood cells, cultured organism antibiotic sensitivity.
- Pyelonephritis:
  - Blood tests (see Table 8.5):
    - FBC: ↑ WCC (infection)
    - U&Es: ↑ urea and creatinine (renal function, dehydration)
    - Glucose: may be ↑ in diabetics
    - CRP: ↑
    - Blood cultures
  - Imaging:
    - USS: stones, obstruction, hydronephrosis
    - X-ray kidneys, ureters and bladder (KUB): stones, soft tissue mass
    - CT-KUB is gold standard investigation for renal tract calculi

> **MICRO-facts**
>
> Infection plus obstruction is a urological emergency!

Table 8.5 Laboratory findings of a urine infection

TEST	CYSTITIS	ACUTE URETHRAL SYNDROME	PYELONEPHRITIS	COMPLICATED UTI
WCC	+++	−/+	+/++	−/+++
Bacterial count	>10^5/mL	Negative	>10^4/mL	Variable
Likely pathogen	• *E. coli* • *Proteus mirabilis* • *Klebsiella* spp. • *Staphylococcus saprophyticus*	• Negative	• *E. coli*	• *E. coli* • *Proteus* spp. • Multi-resistant bacteria • *Mycobacterium tuberculosis* • *Candida* spp.

Emergency and acute medicine

Management

- Upper UTI (pyelonephritis):
  - Analgesia: see Section 1.3
  - IV fluids: 3 L/24 h
  - IV antibiotics: e.g. co-amoxiclav or cefuroxime
  - Admit patient:
    - Monitor fluid balance
    - Investigate underlying cause
- Lower UTI (female, uncomplicated):
  - Discharge with antibiotics: e.g. trimethoprim or amoxicillin for 3–5 days
  - Advise:
    - Drink water regularly
    - Double micturition
    - Void after sexual intercourse
- Lower UTI (male, complicated female):
  - As above, but refer to urology for investigation

Complications

- Septicaemia
- Renal abscess
- Acute kidney injury
- In pregnancy: premature labour
- Uncomplicated UTI → pyelonephritis

MICRO-print

Diagnosis of bacteriuria

In symptomatic patients:
>10^2 coliform organisms/mL urine plus pyuria (>10 WCC/mm³)
OR
>10^5 any pathogenic organisms/mL urine
OR
Any growth of pathogenic organisms in urine by suprapubic aspiration
In asymptomatic patients:
>10^5 pathogenic organisms/MSU urine × 2 occasions

MICRO-case

A 29-year-old female is brought to the ED by her concerned boyfriend as she has vomited four times in the last 24 h, has a fever and rigors. She has a 3-day history of right lower abdominal pain, back pain and dysuria. On exam she has tenderness in her right loin. Urine dipstick was performed while urine was sent for microscopy, culture and sensitivity. Urine dipstick was positive for blood, nitrites and leucocytes. The patient was admitted, urine and blood cultures were taken and she was given IV co-amoxiclav, pain relief, anti-emetics and IV fluids to maintain hydration before starting on oral fluids 8 h later. The patient was sent for a renal USS and KUB plain radiograph which did not show any structural abnormalities along the urinary tract. The results of the MSU showed *E. coli* in the urine, sensitive to cefuroxime and co-amoxiclav.

After 48 h, the patient was discharged with a 7-day oral course of co-amoxiclav and advised to rest for 2 weeks and keep well hydrated.

Key points:

- Dysuria, high fever and rigors are typical features of an upper urinary tract infection.
- There can often be a preceding lower UTI that then extends to the upper tract.
- Symptomatic bacteriuria may require admission for parenteral antibiotics and fluids.
- Stones are an important differential diagnosis, as obstruction with infection of the urinary tract can be life threatening.
- Once the patient's vital signs are stable, if there are no signs of systemic illness, and they can tolerate fluids orally, they can be discharged with a course of antibiotics.

Emergency and acute medicine

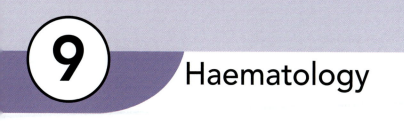

Haematology

9

9.1 ANAEMIA

Definition
- Decreased red blood cell mass, measured by haemoglobin (Hb) concentration:
  - Males: ≤13 g/dL
  - Females: ≤11.5 g/dL

> **MICRO-facts**
>
> Anaemia is commonly an incidental finding following routine full blood count investigation.

Aetiology
- Acute:
  - Frank blood loss
  - Occult blood loss
- Chronic:
  - Chronic disease
  - Inadequate iron absorption or intake
  - Congenital
- Reduced production of red cells, e.g. bone marrow failure
- Increased destruction of erythrocytes, e.g. haemolysis

Clinical features
- General symptoms:
  - Fatigue
  - Weakness
  - Syncope
  - Palpitations
  - Dyspnoea

- Exacerbation of:
  - Asthma
  - COPD
  - Heart failure
  - Angina
- General signs:
  - Pallor
  - Mucous membranes
  - Conjunctiva
  - Palmar creases
  - Tachycardia
  - Orthostatic hypotension
  - Systolic flow murmur (severe)

Diagnostic indicators

- Current/recent trauma: consider acute blood loss
- Recent surgery: consider blood loss
- Gastrointestinal (GI) ulcer: consider occult blood loss
- Weight loss: consider malignancy
- Change in bowel habit: consider malignancy/malabsorption/occult blood loss
- Menorrhagia
- Pregnancy: consider anaemia of pregnancy
- Known chronic inflammatory disease
- Known congenital disorder, e.g. thalassaemia
- Autoimmune disease: consider B_{12} deficiency or anaemia of chronic disease
- Alcohol history: consider folate deficiency
- Mechanical heart valve: consider haemolysis
- Bruising and systemic symptoms: consider bone marrow pathology
- Drug history:
  - NSAIDs: consider GI bleed
  - Methotrexate: consider folate deficiency
- Anticonvulsants: consider folate deficiency

Investigations

- Bloods:
  - FBC – including mean cell volume (MCV)
  - Blood film
  - Iron
  - Ferritin – marker of iron stores; therefore low in iron deficiency
  - Total iron binding capacity (TIBC)
  - Reticulocyte count – immature red cells released in response to anaemia
  - Lactate dehydrogenase (LDH), haptoglobins and direct Coombs to exclude haemolysis

- Serum B_{12} and folate
- U&E – chronic renal failure may lead to anaemia
- Liver function tests – patients with liver disease may have impaired clotting or be prone to varices
- Cross-match (in case transfusion may be required)
- ECG:
  - If cardiac symptoms
  - Check for ischaemic changes

Diagnostic approach
- See Fig. 9.1

Management
- Symptomatic/Hb ≤8 g/dL:
  - Consider transfusion
  - Consult haematology
  - Investigate underlying cause
- Asymptomatic:
  - Treat using iron/folate/B_{12} supplements as appropriate
  - Investigate the underlying cause/refer to speciality or GP
  - Educate about dietary intake

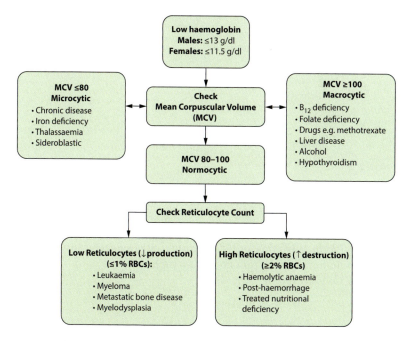

Fig. 9.1 Differential diagnosis of anaemia.

9.2 COAGULOPATHIES

Aetiology

- Congenital:
    - Haemophilia A
    - Haemophilia B
    - Von Willebrand disease
- Acquired:
    - Drug induced: e.g. NSAIDs, steroids, other anticoagulants
    - Disseminated intravascular coagulation (DIC)
    - Liver disease (both acute and chronic)
    - Hypothermia

MICRO-facts

Contact a haematologist when treating somebody with a known bleeding disorder.

Clinical features

- Excessive bleeding relative to injury
- Spontaneous haemorrhage from multiple/uninjured sites:
    - Haemophilia A/B:
        - Large joints (haemarthrosis)
        - Urinary tract
        - Deep muscles
    - Von Willebrand:
        - Epistaxis
        - Gums
        - Menorrhagia

Investigations

- Bloods:
    - FBC: beware that Hb may not adjust for several hours after an acute bleed
    - Clotting screen including:
        - Prothrombin time or INR: measure anticoagulant control
        - Activated partial thromboplastin time (APTT)
        - Consider specific factor levels

Management

- Warfarin control: see Section 9.3
- Wound/fracture:
  - Treat as normal
  - Discuss need for factor replenishment with haematology
- Head trauma/headache/neurological signs:
  - Seek haematology advice
  - CT scan to rule out intracranial haemorrhage

9.3 ANTICOAGULANTS: WARFARIN

Warfarin in the ED

- Initiation following acute thrombosis e.g. DVT/PE
- Assessment of patient concurrently taking warfarin

Considerations

- Many medical drugs and herbal remedies interfere with warfarin/INR measurements
- Check Appendix 1 of the BNF for details before prescribing
- Drugs commonly prescribed in the ED which are known to interact with warfarin include:
  - Antibiotics e.g. clarithromycin
  - Antiepileptics e.g. carbamazepine

MICRO-facts

A patient's condition may also affect warfarin control:
- e.g. Infection
- Alcohol consumption
- Liver disease

Initiation following acute thrombosis

- Check INR:
  - Before giving first dose
  - Every day for 4 days to assess stability
- See local guidelines for loading and maintenance doses.

MICRO-facts

- Warfarin is initially pro-thrombotic.
- Give low molecular weight heparin until 2 days after therapeutic range is reached.

Emergency and acute medicine

Routine monitoring

- Measure INR
- Check value against patient's expected range
- If unknown, check against local/national guidelines (Table 9.1)

> **MICRO-facts**
>
> Patients with prosthetic tissue heart valves generally do not require warfarin except during the first 3 months post surgery.

Table 9.1 **Target INR level in patients taking warfarin, according to condition**

INDICATION	TARGET INR
DVT/PE	2–3
Thrombophilia	2–3
Paroxysmal nocturnal haemaglobinuria (PNH)	2–3
Atrial fibrillation/cardiac emboli	2–3
Mechanical aortic valve	2–3
Mechanical mitral valve	2.5–3.5

Overtreatment
Clinical features

- ↑ INR on routine blood test
- Bleeding
- Anaemia
- Cardiac instability

Management

- Check INR
- Follow algorithm (Fig. 9.2)

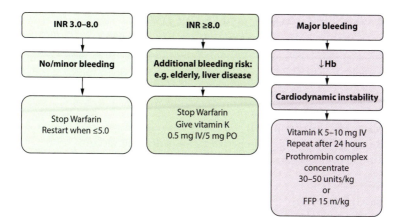

Fig. 9.2 Management of over-treatment with warfarin.

MICRO-case

A 75-year-old man presents to the ED with a productive cough. As part of your routine history, you discover that he takes warfarin for atrial fibrillation. Unfortunately, he does not have his warfarin book with him. On examination, he has a temperature of 38°C and you hear coarse crepitations over his right lung. You order a full blood count, CRP and a chest X-ray. You also include a clotting screen to check his INR. His Hb is normal, but WCC shows leucocytosis. He has a raised CRP and his chest X-ray shows consolidation in the right middle lobe. You diagnose him with pneumonia and wish to start him on antibiotics; however his INR is 4.5 and you are concerned that antibiotics will interfere with this further. You therefore contact haematology, who advise you on what to do next and arrange more frequent INR monitoring.

Key points:
- Always obtain a detailed drug history.
- Ask about warfarin in anybody with one of the following:
  - History of clots or embolic events
  - Atrial fibrillation
  - Valve replacement
- Infection can interfere with warfarin control.
- Many drugs prescribed in the ED, including antibiotics, interfere with warfarin control.
- Prescribing in patients on warfarin is a balancing act, which varies from patient to patient. Always seek advice from haematology/seniors to ensure best practice.

Emergency and acute medicine

9.4 ANTICOAGULANTS: LOW MOLECULAR WEIGHT HEPARIN

Indications

- Deep vein thrombosis (DVT)
- Pulmonary embolism (PE)
- Myocardial infarction (MI)
- Bridging therapy, e.g. peri-operatively for patient on warfarin
- Thromboembolic prophylaxis in the majority of inpatients

Contraindications

- Bleeding disorders
- Recent cerebral haemorrhage
- Peptic ulcer
- Severe hypertension
- eGFR <30

Preparations

- Given subcutaneously
- Check local guidelines or contact pharmacy for preparation stocked:
  - Enoxaparin/Clexane®
  - Dalteparin/Fragmin®
  - Tinzaparin/Innohep®

Complications

- Haemorrhage:
  - Its long half-life and administration route limit the effectiveness of reversal agents
  - Discuss with haematology if major bleeding
- Heparin-induced thrombocytopaenia (<0.5% risk):
  - Check platelet count before initiating therapy
  - Monitor for ↓ platelet count: a fall of 50% should be investigated
  - Combination of arterial and venous thrombosis
- Seek senior help if concerned

9.5 ANTICOAGULANTS: UNFRACTIONATED HEPARIN

Indications

- As for LMW heparin
- Used in patients with eGFR <30
- Patients with high risk of bleeding, as it is reversible and has a short half-life

Contraindications

- Bleeding disorders
- Recent cerebral haemorrhage
- Peptic ulcer
- Severe hypertension

Preparation

- Given as a continuous IV infusion

Complications

- Requires frequent monitoring of APTT and dose adjustment
- Haemorrhage:
  - Stopping the infusion usually suffices
  - Protamine can be administered to reverse the anticoagulant effect – only under specialist supervision
- Heparin-induced thrombocytopaenia:
  - See above, but more common with unfractionated heparin than with LMWH

9.6 ANTICOAGULANTS: OTHER AGENTS

Indications

- As alternatives to warfarin and heparin
- Currently include:
  - Direct thrombin inhibitors, e.g. dabigatran, argatroban
  - Direct factor Xa inhibitors, e.g. rivaroxaban
- Oral preparations recently recommended by NICE for anticoagulation in atrial fibrillation, and DVT prophylaxis post joint replacement
- Therapeutic monitoring not required

Contraindications

- Bleeding disorders
- Recent cerebral haemorrhage
- Peptic ulcer
- Severe hypertension
- Moderate/severe renal impairment

Preparations

- Oral preparations (dabigatran and rivaroxaban), IV preparation (argatroban)

Complications

- Haemorrhage:
  - There is no current specific reversal agent to these therapies
  - Contact haematologist urgently if a patient presents with bleeding while taking these drugs

9.7 BLOOD TRANSFUSION

General principles

- In emergency: transfuse type O rhesus –ve blood or type-specific blood
- If blood may be required later, order:
  - Group and screen:
    - ABO blood group
    - Rhesus D group
  - Cross-match:
    - Full compatibility screen, including antibodies
- Only transfuse if absolutely necessary as per national and local guidelines

Blood products

- See Table 9.2

Table 9.2 **Blood products and indications for their use**

PRODUCT	INDICATION
Packed red cells	Symptomatic/severe anaemia Haemorrhage
Platelets	Symptomatic thrombocytopaenia Platelet dysfunction
Fresh frozen plasma (FFP)	Depletion of multiple coagulation factors: Severe haemorrhage Sepsis Disseminated intravascular coagulation (DIC) Dilutional anaemia Thrombotic thrombocytopaenic purpura (TTP) Haemolytic uraemic syndrome (HUS) Liver disease
Cryoprecipitate (fibrinogen, vWF, VIII, XII)	Massive haemorrhage Factor VII deficiency Von Willebrand disease Hypofibrinogenaemia
Factor VIII concentrate	Factor VIII deficiency (haemophilia A)
Factor IX concentrate	Factor XI deficiency (haemophilia B)

Administration

- See Fig. 9.3

Initial Checks
- Must be performed by **2 members** of staff
- Do not transfuse if **any** discrepancy
- Repeat these checks for every product
    1. Check product expiry date (Figure 9.4 for orientation)
    2. Check product for any lumps/discolouration
    3. Record patient's temperature, pulse and blood pressure before transfusion
    4. Check ID details match those on patient's wrist band
    5. Check ID details match those on the compatibility label
    6. Ensure product prescribed by a doctor
    7. Sign the compatibility form

Delivery
- Transfuse entire bag of blood product
- Infuse via a giving-set with integral filter (to trap aggregates)
- Do not give through a set previously used for anything other than normal saline
- Do not add drugs to a transfusion
- Once started, peel off and return the signed part of the compatibility form

Observation
- Figure 9.5 staff at ALL times
- Record blood pressure, pulse and temperature
    - At start of transfusion
    - 15 minutes into transfusion
- Monitor closely, especially in first 5–10 minutes

If An Adverse Reaction Is Suspected
- Stop transfusion IMMEDIATELY!
- Call for senior help
- Keep IV cannula open with normal saline
- Record vital signs, including urine output
- Re-check patient ID against blood product information
- See 'Transfusion Reaction Algorithm', Figure 9.5

Completion
- Record patient's vital signs
- Document volume of blood transfused
- Change giving set if further fluids are to be administered

Fig. 9.3 Administration of a blood transfusion.

Emergency and acute medicine

Blood transfusion

- See Fig. 9.4

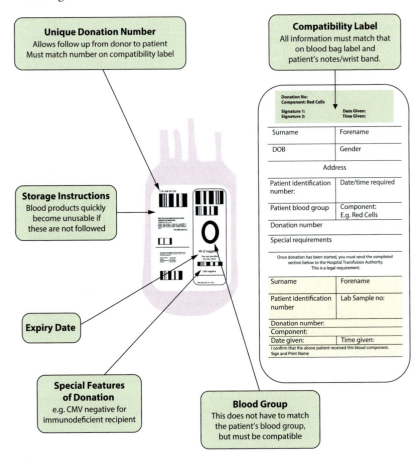

Unique Donation Number
Allows follow up from donor to patient
Must match number on compatibility label

Compatibility Label
All information must match that
on blood bag label and
patient's notes/wrist band.

Storage Instructions
Blood products quickly
become unusable if
these are not followed

Expiry Date

**Special Features
of Donation**
e.g. CMV negative for
immunodeficient recipient

Blood Group
This does not have to match
the patient's blood group,
but must be compatible

Fig. 9.4 Blood transfusion orientation.

Acute blood transfusion reaction

● See Fig. 9.5

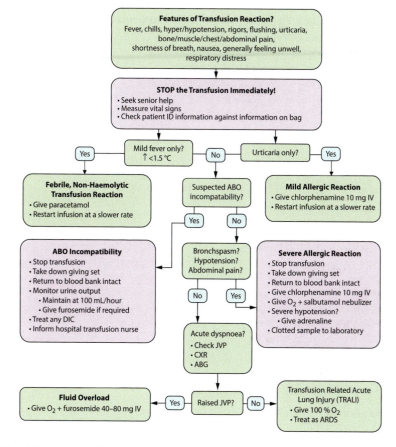

Features of Transfusion Reaction?
Fever, chills, hyper/hypotension, rigors, flushing, urticaria,
bone/muscle/chest/abdominal pain,
shortness of breath, nausea, generally feeling unwell,
respiratory distress

STOP the Transfusion Immediately!
• Seek senior help
• Measure vital signs
• Check patient ID information against information on bag

Mild fever only?
↑ <1.5 °C   No   Urticaria only?   Yes

Yes

**Febrile, Non-Haemolytic
Transfusion Reaction**
• Give paracetamol
• Restart infusion at a slower rate

Suspected ABO
incompatability?

Yes   No

Mild Allergic Reaction
• Give chlorphenamine 10 mg IV
• Restart infusion at a slower rate

ABO Incompatibility
• Stop transfusion
• Take down giving set
• Return to blood bank intact
• Monitor urine output
   • Maintain at 100 mL/hour
   • Give furosemide if required
• Treat any DIC
• Inform hospital transfusion nurse

Bronchspasm?
Hypotension?
Abdominal pain?

No   Yes

Severe Allergic Reaction
• Stop transfusion
• Take down giving set
• Return to blood bank intact
• Give chlorphenamine 10 mg IV
• Give O₂ + salbutamol nebulizer
• Severe hypotension?
   • Give adrenaline
• Clotted sample to laboratory

Acute dyspnoea?
• Check JVP
• CXR
• ABG

Fluid Overload
• Give O₂ + furosemide 40–80 mg IV

Yes   Raised JVP?   No

Transfusion Related Acute
Lung Injury (TRALI)
• Give 100 % O₂
• Treat as ARDS

Fig. 9.5 Acute transfusion reaction algorithm.

9.8 DISSEMINATED INTRAVASCULAR COAGULATION (DIC)

Definition

● Two simultaneous processes:
   ◦ Uncontrolled plasmin release → uncontrolled intravascular coagulation
   ◦ Depletion of platelets/coagulation factors/fibrinogen → haemorrhage

Emergency and acute medicine

Aetiology

- Disorder secondary to other pathology
- Important causes ('MOIST'):
  - **M**alignancy, e.g. acute promyelocytic leukaemia
  - **O**bstetric complications
  - **I**nfection, e.g. meningococcal septicaemia
  - **S**hock, e.g. incompatible transfusion
  - **T**rauma

Clinical features

- Neurological:
  - Delirium
  - Seizure
  - Coma
- Skin:
  - Petechiae
  - Haematoma
- Renal:
  - Oliguria
  - Haematuria

Investigations

- Bloods:
  - FBC: ↓ platelets
  - Clotting screen:
    - INR ↑
    - APTT ↑
    - Fibrinogen ↓ (may be normal initially)

Management

- Control primary cause
- Seek urgent advice from haematology
- Consider replacement of:
  - Platelets
  - Coagulation factors
  - Blood

10 Poisoning and environmental accidents

10.1 ASSESSMENT

ABCDE
- See Chapter 1.
- History/poison not always initially available: look for clues in pockets, witnesses, examination.
- Look for patterns of signs and symptoms suggestive of a toxidrome – e.g. pinpoint pupils, reduced conscious level, and respiratory rate suggests opiate toxicity.

Toxbase®
- National poisons information service.
- Extremely useful information on clinical features and management.
- Medicines information within local hospitals can also access programmes to help identify unknown tablets.

> **MICRO-reference**
> Toxbase: National Poisons Information Service, http://www.toxbase.org/

10.2 PARACETAMOL TOXICITY

Definition
- Significant overdose: 150 mg/kg or 12 g (24 tablets) carries moderate to high risk

Risk factors
- Enzyme-inducing drugs:
  - Phenytoin
  - Carbamazepine

- Rifampicin
- Sulphonylureas
  - Chronic alcohol excess
  - Intercurrent infection
  - Malnourishment:
    - Anorexia
    - Alcoholism
    - Cystic fibrosis
    - HIV

Risk assessment

- Time of ingestion:
  - Triangulate time using:
    - Witness information
    - Mobile phone call/text times
  - If in doubt take the time as the earliest it could be
- Suicide note
- Staggered overdose
- Other drugs ingested
- Alcohol use:
  - Chronic excess ↑ risk of toxicity
  - Acute consumption may be protective

Clinical features

- Within 24 h:
  - Nausea, vomiting
  - Abdominal pain
- >2 days:
  - Jaundice
- >4 days:
  - Hepatic encephalopathy
  - DIC

MICRO-facts

Beware of staggered overdoses!

Investigations

- Paracetamol levels:
  - Take at 4 h post-ingestion.
  - Take as soon as possible if ingestion >4 h ago.

- Use treatment graph (Fig. 10.1) to assess risk of liver damage:
  - Normal treatment line
  - High-risk treatment line
  - With risk factors indicated above
- Other bloods:
  - U&E, bicarbonate
  - LFTs
  - Glucose
  - Venous pH
  - Clotting screen

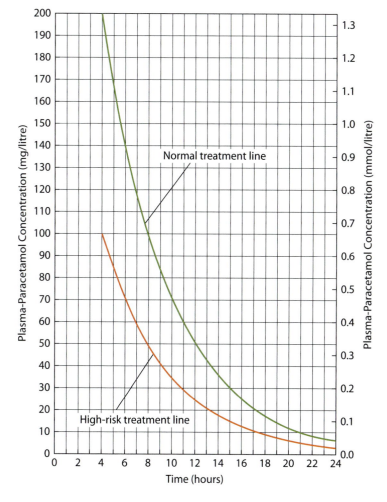

Fig. 10.1 Treatment chart for acetylcysteine in paracetamol.

Management

- Follow treatment outline in Table 10.1
- In staggered overdoses:
  - Start treatment immediately
  - Use the time of first ingestion as the reference point for placing paracetamol level on the treatment graph
- Psychiatric review before discharge

Table 10.1 **Management of paracetamol overdose**

TIME POST-INGESTION	MANAGEMENT
<1 h	Activate charcoal if >12 g ingested

0–8 h	Check plasma paracetamol at 4 h
	If above treatment line on graph start treatment
	IV N-acetylcysteine in following order:
	    150 mg/kg in 200 mL dextrose over 15 min
	    50 mg/kg in 500 mL dextrose over 4 h
	    100 mg/kg in 1000 mL dextrose over 16 h
	Oral methionine:
	    Used if N-acetylcysteine not available
	    2.5 g every 4 h to a total of 10 g

8–15 h	Start N-acetylcysteine if >12 g paracetamol ingested Do not wait for plasma paracetamol levels
15–24 h	Urgent N-acetylcysteine Late presentation has severe risk Check plasma paracetamol level, renal function, LFTs, prothrombin time, pH Assess for signs of encephalopathy
>24 h	If >12 g paracetamol ingested start N-acetylcysteine Seek expert advice

MICRO-print
- N-acetylcysteine (NAC) can cause anaphylactoid reactions.
- Treat with antihistamines, fluids, supportive care (see Chapter 1); slow the rate of infusion.

10.3 ASPIRIN TOXICITY

Clinical features
- Vomiting
- Tinnitus
- Hyperventilation
- Confusion
- Mixed metabolic acidosis and respiratory alkalosis

Investigations
- Bloods:
  - U&E:
    - Electrolyte abnormalities
    - Acute renal failure
  - ABG:
    - Mixed respiratory alkalosis and metabolic acidosis
  - Glucose

Management
- Activated charcoal:
  - Within 1 h of ingestion and >120 mg/kg
- Consider sodium bicarbonate if:
  - Metabolic acidosis
  - Salicylate levels >500 mg/L
  - Patient may need to be observed in ITU
- Haemodialysis if:
  - Patient unresponsive to above measures
  - CNS features are present
  - Salicylate levels >700 mg/L
- Psychiatric review before discharge

10.4 OPIOID TOXICITY

Clinical features
- Venepuncture marks
- Iatrogenic – check inpatient medication charts
- Pinpoint pupils
- ↓ RR
- ↓ GCS
- Evidence of addiction:
  - Multiple venepuncture marks, old and new
  - Thrombosed veins

Emergency and acute medicine

Investigations

- Bloods:
  - FBC
  - U&Es: poor renal function can exacerbate toxicity
  - LFTs
  - Clotting screen
  - Glucose: rule out hypoglycaemia
  - Other drug levels:
    - Paracetamol
    - Salicylates
- ABG: type II respiratory failure
- ECG: may show runs of VT
- Urine toxicology: opioid positive
- CXR: high risk of aspiration

Management

- ABCDE: assisted ventilation with bag and mask
- Exclude organic illness/injury, e.g. hypoglycaemia, head injury, infection
- Naloxone:
  - 0.4–0.8 mg IV every 2 min – maximum 1.2 mg
  - Titrate dose according to response
  - Give dose IM as well as IV, to prolong effect of naloxone, and if struggling with IV access
  - Shorter half-life than opioids, symptoms of toxicity can recur
  - Consider naloxone infusion 0.1–0.4 mg/h if still symptomatic
  - Observe for 6 h after last dose; long-acting opioids naturally have a longer half-life and so will require longer observation. See Toxbase for advice with individual preparations
  - Respiratory depression, coma may recur
- Avoid fully reversing opioid in addicts
- Nurse in left lateral position to reduce the risk of aspiration
- Risk assessment: psychiatric management of the patient (if necessary)

10.5 TRICYCLIC TOXICITY

Clinical features

- Anticholinergic:
  - Dry skin
  - Urinary retention
  - Dilated pupils

- Neurological:
  - Altered level of consciousness
  - Convulsions
- Cardiovascular:
  - Sinus tachycardia
  - Arrhythmias
  - ECG abnormalities – see below

Investigations

- Bloods:
  - FBC
  - U&E
  - LFTs
  - Prothrombin time (PT)
  - Glucose
  - Blood levels:
    - Paracetamol
    - Salicylates
- ABG:
  - Hypoxia
  - Metabolic acidosis
  - Electrolyte discrepancies
- ECG:
  - Prolonged PR interval
  - Non-specific T wave changes
  - Broad QRS
  - Prolonged QT segment
  - Heart block
  - VT

Management

- ABCDE
- Oral-activated charcoal:
  - If presentation is within 1 h of ingestion
  - Ensure secure airway before administration
- IV fluids
- Sodium bicarbonate for acidosis, broad QRS and arrhythmias
- With significant overdoses, HDU/ITU admission is almost always required
- Psychiatric review before discharge

Emergency and acute medicine

10.6 BENZODIAZEPINE TOXICITY

Clinical features
- CNS depression: ↓ GCS
- Ataxia
- Slurred speech
- Respiratory depression
- Hypotonia
- Coma
- With significant overdoses, HDU/ITU admission is almost always required

Investigations
- Bloods:
  - FBC
  - U&E: assess renal function
  - LFT
  - Clotting screen
  - Glucose: rule out other causes such as hypoglycaemia
- Blood levels: paracetamol and salicylate
- ABG: respiratory acidosis
- ECG

Management
- Respiratory depression:
  - Maintain airway
  - Intubate
  - Assist ventilation, if required
- Monitor frequently:
  - GCS
  - ECG
- Supportive therapy: IV fluids as required
- Consider antidote:
  - Flumazenil
  - Only in iatrogenic benzodiazepine toxicity where it is the only drug taken
- Psychiatric review before discharge

10.7 CARBON MONOXIDE POISONING

Clinical features
- Depends on duration and concentration of CO exposure:
  - May be asymptomatic
  - Headache
  - Breathlessness

- Malaise
- Cognitive impairment
- Cherry-red skin
- Respiratory failure
- Cardiac arrest

> **MICRO-facts**
> - Chronic low concentration exposure → non-specific symptoms
> - Short-duration high-concentration exposure → severe symptoms and metabolic acidosis

Management
- High-flow oxygen
- Consider intubation
- Fluid resuscitation

10.8 OTHER TOXINS AND ANTIDOTES

- See Table 10.2

Table 10.2 **Toxins and antidotes**

TOXIN	ANTIDOTE
Beta-blockers	Glucagon
Digoxin	Digibind®
Iron	Desferrioxamine
Organophosphates	Atropine

10.9 BURNS

Assessment
- History:
  - Circumstance of burn:
    - Enclosed space? (CO poisoning)
    - Duration of exposure to smoke/fire
    - Material that was burning: was it toxic?
- Examination:
  - Hoarse voice
  - Singed nasal hair
  - Restriction in lung expansion

- Exposure, estimation of extent of burn: rule of nines – quick method to estimate body surface burned (see Fig. 10.2 and Table 10.3; see also Table 10.4 for degree of burn calculation)

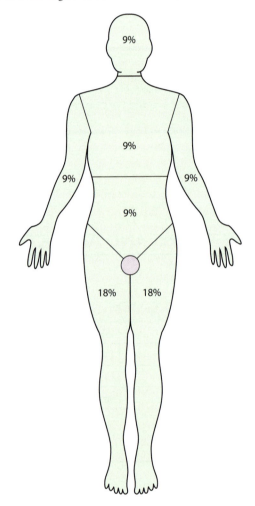

Fig. 10.2 Rule of nines body chart.

Table 10.3 **Rule of nines**

BODY PART	PERCENTAGE
Head	9%
Chest (front)	9%
Abdomen (front)	9%
Back and buttocks	18%
Each arm	9%
Each palm	1%
Groin	1%
Each leg	18%

Management

- A, B:
  - Intubate early if airway involvement likely – it will swell very quickly!
  - Oxygen
  - Be aware that chest burns can restrict lung expansion; may need surgical release – escharotomy
- C:
  - IV fluid resuscitation
  - Aim for a urine output of 1 mL/kg/h as a minimum
  - Analgesia
  - Consider tetanus prophylaxis
  - Monitor potassium:
    - Hyperkalaemia can occur due to muscle damage which can result in acute renal failure
  - Bandaging:
    - Cling film initially
    - Biosynthetic dressings speed up wound healing
  - Antibiotics not routinely given
  - Referral to specialist burns management unit:
    - Burns over 10% children, 15% adults
    - Respiratory burns
    - Face, hands, feet, perineum, genitalia burns
  - Check for secondary infection

Emergency and acute medicine

Table 10.4 **Degree burn developed**

DEGREE BURN	DEPTH	APPEARANCE
Superficial thickness	Epidermis	Erythema, tender
Partial thickness – superficial	Superficial dermis	Blisters
Partial thickness – deep	Deep dermis	Whiter appearance, ↓ sensation
Full thickness	Destruction to subcutaneous fat	Charred, leather, no sensation

---

MICRO-print

Parkland Formula

- This can be used to guide the rate of fluid administration in burns.
- Fluid is administered at 4 mL/kg per body surface area burned.
- First 50% – initial 8 h.
- Second 50% – subsequent 16 h.
- Additional maintenance fluid:
  - 1–1.5 mL/kg/h

MICRO-case

An HIV-positive 25-year-old male presents to ED after taking 30 tablets of paracetamol in a suicide attempt. He took the tablets over a period of 5 h. He is brought to the ED 6 h after the first ingestion.

On arrival patient is alert, but appears anxious and tearful. His partner attends, and explains that she found a note when she returned early from work explaining his reasons for the suicide attempt. She has brought in several empty paracetamol packets, but is unsure if he has taken other drugs or alcohol with it. IV access is obtained, venous gas, FBC, clotting screen, LFTs, U&Es, glucose and plasma paracetamol and salicylate levels are sent immediately. IV N-acetylcysteine is started promptly without waiting for paracetamol levels to return.

Key points:
- The patient has taken 15 g of paracetamol which carries a moderate to severe risk.
- An important point is that the overdose was taken over a 5 h period, and thus the time of the first ingestion should be used as the reference point.
- It is important not to delay treatment, especially as the patient also has HIV, and this will put him at a higher risk. In any case,

continued...

continued...

a paracetamol level result is unlikely to be available before the 8 h watershed when glutathione reserves are exhausted. His plasma paracetamol levels should be taken immediately, as there is no need to wait for 4 h, given that he started the overdose 6 h ago.

- It is important to also test for salicylate levels, as often multiple drugs are used in overdoses.
- A collateral history should be obtained from relatives to obtain further clues about the attempt. Suicide notes often indicate a more serious attempt, and after the patient is medically stable, psychiatric assistance should be sought from the crisis team, who are generally available 24 h a day. See Chapter 19, Psychiatry.

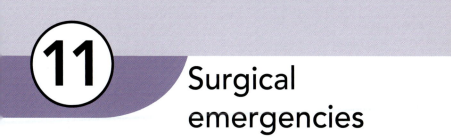

11 Surgical emergencies

11.1 ACUTE ABDOMINAL PAIN

Aetiology
- See Table 11.1

Table 11.1 **Causes of acute abdominal pain**

SURGICAL	GYNAECOLOGICAL	MEDICAL
• Acute appendicitis • Biliary colic • Cholangitis • Acute cholecystitis • Acute pancreatitis • Diverticulitis • Bowel obstruction • Perforation of viscus • Renal calculi • Urinary retention • Testicular torsion • Mesenteric ischaemia • Trauma	• Ectopic pregnancy • Ovarian cyst torsion • Pelvic inflammatory disease • Endometriosis • Dysmenorrhoea • Obstetric pathologies	• Irritable bowel syndrome • Gastroenteritis • Inflammatory bowel disease • Myocardial infarction • Pulmonary embolism • Diabetic ketoacidosis • Urinary tract infection • Pyelonephritis • Lower lobe pneumonia • GORD/gastritis/duodenitis

History
- Nature of pain:
  - Location
  - Onset
  - Character
  - Radiation
  - Severity
  - Aggravating/improving factors
  - Variability and duration

Emergency and acute medicine

- GI symptoms:
  - Diarrhoea
  - Appetite
  - Bloating
  - Constipation
  - Haematemesis/PR bleeding/mucous
  - Weight loss
  - Nausea/vomiting:
    - Character of vomit:
      - Blood
      - Bile
      - Quantity
    - Timing:
      - Prior to pain usually in medical conditions
      - After pain usually in surgical conditions
- Gynaecological symptoms:
  - Last menstrual period: rule out pregnancy
  - Dysmenorrhoea
  - Menorrhagia
  - Intermenstrual bleeding
  - Post-coital bleeding
  - Vaginal discharge
  - Previous pelvic inflammatory disease
  - Sexual history
- Urinary symptoms:
  - Dysuria
  - Urinary frequency/polyuria
  - Haematuria/urinary discolouration
  - Hesitancy/terminal dribbling
  - Urethral discharge
  - Recent catheterization/urological procedure

Examination

- Basic:
  - General appearance
  - Vital signs: blood pressure, heart rate, respiratory rate, oxygen saturations
  - Temperature
  - Urine output
- Abdominal examination
- Hernial orifices

- Palpate the abdominal aorta and the peripheral pulses
- Rectal examination
- Examination of external genitalia if appropriate
- Other systemic examinations

Investigations

- Bloods:
  - FBC: a raised WCC may indicate infection
  - U&E
  - Glucose: DKA can present with abdominal pain
  - LFTs: look for hepatitic vs. obstructive pattern; see MICRO-fact box
  - Amylase: often elevated in pancreatitis
  - Clotting screen
  - Group and save: surgical intervention ± blood transfusion may be required
- Urine dipstick ± MC&S
- Serum or urinary ß-hCG
- ECG: myocardial ischaemia and infarction can also be a cause of abdominal pain
- Radiology:
  - Erect CXR: free gas under the diaphragm may indicate viscus perforation
  - AXR: may show signs of bowel obstruction
  - Abdominal/pelvic ultrasound scans
  - CT scan

MICRO-facts

Hepatic vs. obstructive LFTs
- Hepatic LFTs:
  - Hepatocellular damage results in the release of transaminases
  - ↑AST, ↑ALT
  - Hepatitis, fatty liver, Wilson's disease, drugs
- Obstructive LFTs:
  - Obstruction to bile outflow from the bile duct
  - ↑Bilirubin, ↑ALP, ↑GGT
  - Gallstones, pancreatic cancer, bile duct stricture

11.2 APPENDICITIS

Definition
- Inflammation of the vermiform appendix
- The most common surgical emergency
- Common in all ages

Clinical features
- Abdominal pain:
  - Gradual onset
  - Begins colicky and central
  - Shifts to localize over the right iliac fossa as the visceral peritoneum becomes inflamed
- Nausea and vomiting
- Anorexia
- Low-grade pyrexia
- Tachycardia
- Abdominal guarding on examination and percussion tenderness over the right iliac fossa
  - Presence of Rovsing's sign

MICRO-facts

Clinical signs in appendicitis
- Rosving's sign:
  - Pressure on the left iliac fossa results in pain in the right iliac fossa
- Cope sign:
  - If the appendix is lying close to the obturator internus, flexion and internal rotation of the right hip elicits pain
- Psoas sign:
  - If there is a retrocaecal appendix, extending the hip causes pain

---

Investigation
- Often diagnosed clinically
- Serum or urinary ß-hCG to rule out ectopic pregnancy
- Bloods:
  - FBC: neutrophil leucocytosis
  - U&E
  - LFT

- CRP: ↑
- Group and save
- USS or CT may confirm diagnosis

Management

- Keep nil by mouth
- Analgesia: see Section 1.3
- Antiemetics, e.g. cyclizine 50 mg IV
- Intravenous fluids
- Organize surgical review: consider appendicectomy

> **MICRO-facts**
>
> Gallstones are the most common cause of biliary tract disease. Exact pathology is dependent on the site of the stone.

11.3 GALLSTONES

Definition

- Hard biliary component deposits that form inside the gallbladder (see Table 11.2)

Table 11.2 **Location of gallstone and condition caused**

GALLBLADDER	INSIDE BILIARY TREE	OUTSIDE BILIARY TREE
• Biliary colic • Acute cholecystitis • Mucocoele • Empyema	• Biliary colic • Ascending cholangitis • Obstructive jaundice • Pancreatitis	• Gallstone ileus

BILIARY COLIC

Definition

- Pain secondary to the passage of gallstones into the biliary tree

Clinical features

- Often known to have gallstones
- Abdominal pain:
  - Right upper quadrant and epigastric region
  - Often referred to the scapula
  - Recurrent
  - Colicky in nature
  - Often occurs after a fatty meal

> **MICRO-facts**
>
> Gallstones common in:
>   **F**air
>   **F**at
>   **F**orty
>   **F**ertile
>   **F**emales

- Vomiting
- Jaundice: if the common bile duct becomes obstructed (see below)

Investigations

- Bloods:
    - FBC – if raised WCC, implies infection, e.g. acute cholecystitis or ascending cholangitis (see below)
    - U&E
    - LFTs – if abnormal, implies obstruction (see below)
    - Amylase
- Abdominal ultrasound scan – to visualize stones within the gallbladder

Management

- Nil by mouth
- Analgesia: see Section 1.3
- IV fluids
- Refer for surgical review
- If pain has subsided:
    - Consider discharge
    - Advise low-fat diet
    - Arrange surgical outpatient follow-up to consider cholecystectomy

ACUTE CHOLECYSTITIS

Definition

- Obstructed gallbladder with infection

Clinical features

- Pain:
    - Right upper quadrant
    - Radiates to the right side of the back/tip of the shoulder
    - Constant
    - Severe
- Vomiting
- Pyrexia

- Right upper quadrant tenderness
- Guarding
- Positive Murphy sign (see MICRO-fact)

> ## MICRO-facts
>
> **Murphy sign**
>
> Pressure over the right upper quadrant (but not over the left upper quadrant) on deep inspiration will cause the patient to catch their breath due to pain, as the diaphragm pushes the inflamed infected gallbladder towards the examining fingers.

Investigations

- Bloods:
    - FBC: ↑ WCC
    - U&E
    - LFTs may be deranged in obstruction
    - Amylase
- Abdominal ultrasound scan: presence of gallstones

Management

- Nil by mouth
- Analgesia: see Section 1.3
- Antiemetic, e.g. cyclizine 50 mg IV, max. 8 hourly
- IV fluids
- IV Antibiotics:
    - E.g. co-amoxiclav 1.2 g twice daily if not penicillin allergic
    - Please check local guidelines as antibiotic prescribing may vary
- Arrange admission and surgical review

OBSTRUCTIVE JAUNDICE

Definition

- Jaundice secondary to bile duct obstruction

Clinical features

- Pale stools
- Dark urine
- Right upper quadrant pain
- Jaundice
- Painless jaundice is a red flag symptom and may indicate obstruction due to malignancy e.g. carcinoma of head of the pancreas

Emergency and acute medicine

> ## MICRO-facts
>
> **Courvoisier's law**
> If the gallbladder is palpable in the presence of obstructive jaundice, the cause is unlikely to be a stone.

Investigations

- Bloods:
    - FBC
    - U&E
    - LFTs
- Raised conjugated bilirubin, ALP, AST, ALT:
    - Amylase
- Pancreatitis can result from gallstones
- Abdominal ultrasound scan to detect presence of gallstones within the common bile duct
- May require MRCP/ERCP as an inpatient

Management

- Referral to surgical team for further investigations

ASCENDING CHOLANGITIS

Definition

- Biliary tree infection secondary to biliary stasis

Clinical features

- Charcot's triad
    - Fever
    - Right upper quadrant pain
    - Jaundice

Investigations

- Bloods:
    - FBC – raised WCC indicates infection
    - U&E
    - LFTs – deranged due to obstruction
    - Amylase – pancreatitis may be concommitant
- Ultrasound scan – to demonstrate the presence of bile duct stones
- AXR; gas in the biliary tree

Management

- Analgesia: see Section 1.3
- IV fluids
- Intravenous antibiotics: see Section 18.2
- Arrange admission and medical/surgical review

ACUTE PANCREATITIS

Definition

- An inflammatory condition of the pancreas

Clinical features

- Pain:
  - Severe
  - Radiates through to the back
  - Eased by leaning forward
- Nausea and vomiting
- Mild pyrexia
- Dehydration/shock:
  - Tachycardia
  - Hypotension
- Jaundice
- Epigastric tenderness and guarding

MICRO-facts

Causes of acute pancreatitis: GET SMASHED

Gallstones
Ethanol
Trauma
Steroids
Mumps
Automimmune
Scorpion venom
Hyperlipidaemia, hypercalcaemia, hypothermia
ERCP
Drugs – thiazide diuretics

Investigations

- See Table 11.3.

Table 11.3 Investigation findings in acute pancreatitis

INVESTIGATION	FINDINGS
FBC	↑ WCC
U&E	Renal failure: ↑ urea/↑ creatinine
Glucose	Raised
Amylase	Level >1000 confirms diagnosis
C-reactive protein	Indicates severity of attack: >150 in first 48 h is severe
LFTs	↑ Bilirubin confirms presence of jaundice Raised AST indicates severity
Calcium	Hypocalcaemia
ABG	↓ PaO_2 and lactate can indicate severity
Erect chest X-ray	Excludes viscus perforation and pneumonia
Abdominal X-ray	Calcification around the head of pancreas
Abdominal ultrasound scan	Inflammation of pancreas
	Presence of gallstones
	Dilated bile ducts
CT scan	May identify haemorrhage and necrosis of pancreas
ECG	Exclude myocardial infarction

Prognostic indicators

- See MICRO-fact: 'Glasgow Criteria'.

Management

- Oxygen: if low PaO_2
- Nil by mouth: avoid stimulating the pancreas; consider nasogastric tube if vomiting
- IV fluids
- Analgesia: see Section 1.3
- Antiemetic, e.g. metoclopramide 10 mg, max.; 8 hourly
- Urinary catheter: urine output monitoring
- Consider HDU or ITU in severe cases
- Refer for urgent surgical review

> ### MICRO-facts
>
> **Glasgow criteria**
>
> The presence of three or more criteria within 48 h indicates severe acute pancreatitis.
>
> | | |
> |---|---|
> | **P** | **p**O_2 <7.9 kPa |
> | **A** | **A**ge >55 years |
> | **N** | **N**eutrophils >15 × 10^9/L |
> | **C** | **C**alcium <2 mmol/L |
> | **R** | **R**aised urea >16 mmol/L |
> | **E** | **E**nzymes – LDH >600 U/L/AST >100 U/L |
> | **A** | **A**lbumin <32 g/L |
> | **S** | **S**ugar – glucose >10 mmol/L |

> **MICRO-print**
> Dehydration and hypotension can be severe in acute pancreatitis. Hypotension results from third space losses and the release of vasoactive mediators in pancreatic exudate that have an effect on the myocardium and vascular tone. Such patients therefore may require inotropic support in a critical care environment, so consider early critical care review to reduce mortality.

11.4 ACUTE BOWEL OBSTRUCTION

Causes

- See Table 11.4

Table 11.4 **Causes of bowel obstruction**

MECHANICAL	NON-MECHANICAL (PARALYTIC ILEUS)
Carcinoma	Post-operative
Obstructed hernia	Electrolyte abnormalities
Adhesions from previous surgery	Hypokalaemia, hypomagnesaemia
Gallstones	Medication – anticholinergics
Intussusception	Hypothyroidism
Ingested foreign body	

Emergency and acute medicine

Clinical features

- Abdominal distension: more noticeable with large bowel obstruction
- Abdominal pain:
  - Central
  - Colicky
  - Severe pain may suggest strangulation with resulting bowel ischaemia
- Vomiting: occurs early in small bowel obstruction
- Absolute constipation:
  - No faeces
  - No flatus
- Dehydration/signs of shock:
  - Reduced BP
  - ↑ HR
- Low-grade pyrexia
- Abdominal examination:
  - Distended tender tympanic abdomen
  - Tinkling bowel sounds in mechanical obstruction
  - No bowel sounds in paralytic ileus
  - Scars from previous surgery
  - Examine hernial orifices: check for strangulated herniae
- Rectal examination: often an empty rectum is found

Investigations

- FBC: leucocytosis may be present
- U&Es: may reveal electrolyte abnormality
- Group and save: in case surgery is required
- Erect CXR: gas under the diaphragm may indicate perforation
- AXR: dilated bowel loops (see Table 11.5)
- See Fig. 11.1 and 11.2

Table 11.5 **Radiographic differences between small and large bowel obstruction**

SMALL BOWEL OBSTRUCTION	LARGE BOWEL OBSTRUCTION
Dilated bowel loops are central	Dilated bowel loops are peripheral
Small-diameter loops of bowel (3.5 cm)	Large-diameter loops of bowel (5.5 cm; caecum is 8 cm)
Valvulae conniventes are small white lines that are visible all the way across the section of the bowel	Haustrae are thick lines that partially cross the bowel

Management

- Nil by mouth
- Intravenous fluids
- Analgesia: see Section 1.3

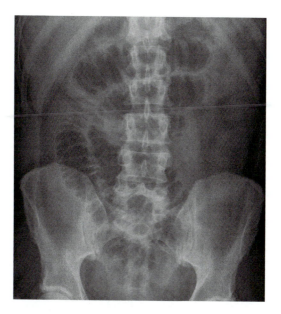

Fig. 11.1 Small bowel obstruction. (From Fig. 6.4a from Lisle, *Imaging for Students*, 3rd ed., CRC Press, Boca Raton, FL, 2007, pp. 94, 95.)

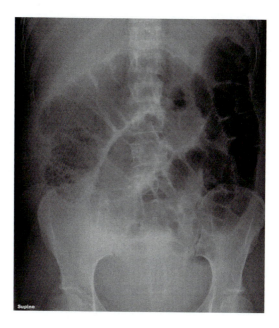

Fig. 11.2 Large bowel obstruction. (From Fig. 6.5a from Lisle, *Imaging for Students*, 3rd ed., CRC Press, Boca Raton, FL, 2007, pp. 94, 95.)

- Urinary catheter: monitor fluid balance
- Nasogastric tube:
  - Prevents vomiting
  - Relieves pressure
  - Prevents aspiration
- Refer for surgical review

MICRO-case

An 85-year-old male with a history of gallstones was admitted to the surgical ward with severe right upper quadrant pain. During the night he has faeculent vomiting and appears unwell. On questioning, he states he has not opened his bowels for 7 days and is not passing flatus.

On examination he has a distended tympanic abdomen with quiet bowel sounds. His urine output has only been 700 mL in the last 24 h.

An AXR shows central dilated bowel loops.

This patient will need to be kept nil by mouth, a nasogastric tube will need to be inserted. Adequate IV fluids will need to be given, and a catheter will need to be inserted so that strict fluid monitoring can take place. Antiemetics and analgesia will need to be given intravenously and urgent surgical review is required for further management.

Key Points:
- This patient has a history of gallstones and it appears that the gallstones have left the biliary system and entered the gastrointestinal tract via the duodenum resulting in acute bowel obstruction, or **gallstone ileus**.
- This is a rare condition but an important differential to remember.
- Treatment is as per small bowel obstruction.

11.5 MESENTERIC INFARCTION

Definition
- Reduced intestinal blood flow
- Reduction or cessation of blood flow results in acute mesenteric ischaemia/infarction

Aetiology
- See Table 11.6

Table 11.6 **Aetiology of mesenteric infarction**

AETIOLOGY	FEATURES
Embolism	Associated with atrial fibrillation
Thrombosis	Pre-existing atherosclerosis
Other causes	Hypotension Intestinal vasospasm

Clinical features

- Elderly patients
- Abdominal pain:
  - Diffuse
  - Severe
  - Disproportionate to clinical abdominal examination findings
- Bloody diarrhoea
- Vomiting
- Shock
  - ↑ HR
  - ↓ BP
- Abdominal examination:
  - Tenderness
  - Distension
  - Absent bowel sounds

Management

- IV access
- Bloods:
  - FBC
  - U&E
  - Clotting screen
  - Cross-match
- ABG: metabolic acidosis/↑ lactate
- IV fluid resuscitation
- Analgesia: see Section 1.3
- IV antibiotics dependent on local guidelines
- NGT
- Refer for urgent surgical review; CT/angiography confirm diagnosis

11.6 UROLOGY

RENAL COLIC

Definition

- Calculi present in the renal tract
- 75% of calculi consist of calcium oxalate

Risk factors

- Males:females – 2:1
- Hypercalcaemia
- Hyperuricaemia
- Dehydration

- UTIs
- Thiazide diuretics

> ### MICRO-facts
>
> In men over 50 years old, always consider a leaking abdominal aortic aneurysm as a differential diagnosis.

Clinical features

- Severe pain:
    - Typically loin to groin
    - Constant dull ache with episodes of severe colicky pain
    - Unable to find a comfortable position
- Haematuria: due to damage to the renal tract epithelium by the calculi
- Pyrexia
- Nausea

Investigations

- See Table 11.7

Table 11.7 **Investigation findings in renal colic**

INVESTIGATION	FINDINGS
FBC	• ↑ WCC
U&E	• Assess renal function • ↑ urea and creatinine in acute kidney injury
Calcium Magnesium Phosphate Uric acid	• May give an indication of the type of stone
KUB X-ray (kidneys, ureter, bladder)	• 60% of calculi are radio-opaque
CT KUB scan	• 95% sensitive • Detects other pathology including AAA
Urine dipstick	• Haematuria

Management

- Analgesia:
    - Morphine 1–10 mg IV titrate according to pain
    - Diclofenac 100 mg PR
- Antiemetic e.g. metoclopramide 10 mg, max. 8 hourly
- Intravenous fluids

- Admit patients with:
  - Urinary tract infection
  - Persistent pain
  - Renal impairment
  - Obstructed kidney
- Refer to urology for review and further investigation
- Systemically well patients with normal renal function and only mild haematuria on urine dipstick, in whom pain has resolved, may be discharged with urology outpatient follow-up

> ## MICRO-facts
>
> Fever + raised WCC + obstructed kidney = infected obstructed kidney
> This is a surgical emergency. The patient will need IV antibiotics and a nephrostomy tube insertion.

TESTICULAR TORSION

See also Chapter 14, Paediatrics.

Definition

- Twisting of the spermatic cord which compromises the blood supply to the testicle
- Can cause necrosis due to vascular compromise of the testicle
- Common in children around puberty

Clinical features

- Abdominal pain
- Acute scrotal pain
- Vomiting
- Testicular examination: erythematous, high riding, exquisitely tender, swollen testicle which may be lying horizontally in its long axis
- Difficulty walking due to pain

Investigations

- Scrotal Doppler ultrasound: compromised blood flow to the affected testicle often with concurrent reactive hydrocoele

Management

- Analgesia: see Section 1.3
- Keep nil by mouth
- Urgent surgical review: will require exploration under anaesthesia ideally within 6 h of symptom onset in order to prevent irreversible testicular damage
- If torted, the other testicle will be fixed at the same time to prevent recurrence in this testicle

Emergency and acute medicine

MICRO-facts

Torsion of the cyst of Morgagni may mimic testicular torsion and may be difficult to differentiate on clinical examination. Sometimes a small tender purple nodule may be evident to the scrotal sac which is the torted cyst.

TESTICULAR LUMPS

Aetiology

- Infective: orchitis/epididymo-orchitis:
  - Mumps
  - STI
  - Ascending urinary tract infections
- See Fig. 11.3

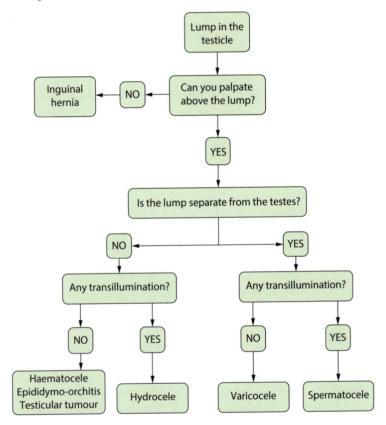

Fig. 11.3 Aetiology of testicular lumps.

ORCHITIS/EPIDIDYMO-ORCHITIS

Clinical features

- Tender, swollen testicle/epididymis
- Systemic upset
- Urethral discharge

Investigation

- MSU for dipstick and MC&S
- Urethral swab
- Mumps serology

Management

- Antibiotics, e.g. ciprofloxacin 500 mg twice daily for 10–14 days
- Analgesia
- Scrotal support
- GUM clinic follow-up with contact tracing if STD confirmed

11.7 VASCULAR

ABDOMINAL AORTIC ANEURYSM

Definition

- A localized dilatation of the abdominal aorta resulting in weakening of the muscular vascular wall

Risk factors

- Usually over 65 years
- More common in males
- Systemic atherosclerotic disease

Clinical features

- Pain:
    - Epigastric, back or flank
    - Often radiates to the groin
    - Sudden onset
- Features of shock:
    - Pale
    - Syncope
    - Decreased conscious level
    - Tachycardia
    - Hypotension
    - Abdominal mass: tender, expansile, pulsatile

Emergency and acute medicine

Investigation

- Bloods:
    - FBC
    - U&E
    - Clotting screen
    - Cross match: 6–10 units
- Urgent focussed abdominal aortic assessment ultrasound scan/non-contrast CT scan: confirm diagnosis
- ECG

Management

- Oxygen
- Avoid intravenous fluids: allow permissive hypotension to avoid further bleeding
- Analgesia
- Antiemetic, e.g. metoclopramide 10 mg, max. 8 hourly
- Immediate vascular surgeon and anaesthetist review for urgent operative repair

ACUTE LIMB ISCHAEMIA

Aetiology

- Thrombotic:
    - Most common
    - Previous atheromatous disease
    - Features of chronic vascular insufficiency – muscle wasting, venous eczema, haemosiderosis, hair loss, ulceration
- Embolic:
    - Emboli lodge in the vascular system
    - 80% of emboli are from AF; the rest are from atheromatous disease
    - Faster onset of symptoms

Clinical features

- The '6 Ps':
    - **P**ain
    - **P**allor
    - **P**ulselessness
    - **P**araesthesia
    - **P**aralysis: motor compromise as musculature becomes ischaemic
    - **P**erishingly cold

Management

- Analgesia
- IV fluids
- Heparinization: see Chapter 9, Haematology
- Urgent vascular review for attempted re-vascularization

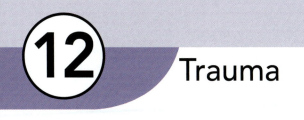

12 Trauma

12.1 RESUSCITATION

Principles

- Resuscitation always follows an ABCDE approach to identify and manage life-threatening injuries
- Continuous reassessment is essential throughout the primary survey
- Return to 'A' for airway, following:
  - A change to condition
  - Any intervention to assess patient response
- Proceed to secondary survey: top to toe, front and back when primary survey complete and patient stabilized and fully alert (having received definitive care, e.g. surgery) which may have to be several days later
- Do not forget to give analgesia to trauma patients in pain

Primary survey

- Work through Fig. 12.1

Secondary survey

- Once life-threatening issues identified
- AMPLE history and mechanism of injury:
  - Allergies
  - Medicines: anticoagulants, insulin and cardiovascular medications
  - Past medical/surgical history/pregnancy
  - Last meal
  - Events/environment surrounding injury i.e. exactly what happened
- Thorough physical examination with investigation and management of other identified injuries

PRIMARY SURVEY

- Airway maintainence with cervical spine protection, collar headblocks and straps: triple immobilization

- 'Breathing and ventilation, ensuring adequate oxygenation'

- Circulation with haemorrhage control; secure adequate venous access with direct pressure to bleeding wounds/use of tourniquets/emergency haemostatic status

- Disability
  - Level of consciousness AVPU/GCS
  - Pupils: size, equality, reactions
  - Glasgow coma scale <8: involve an anaesthetist early to secure and maintain the airway
  - Do not forget glucose

- Exposure with environmental control: to assess all injuries while avoiding hypothermia

- Adjuncts to the primary survey
  - Vital signs: BP, pulse, respiratory rate, oxygen saturations
  - Monitor volume: urinary catheter
  - Plain trauma series radiographs: cervical spine, chest and pelvis
  - However, do not let these adjuncts slow down the primary survey
  - Do not forget adequate analgesia

Fig. 12.1 Primary survey.

MICRO-facts

Take an **AMPLE** history:

A	Allergies
M	Medications
P	Previous medical/surgical history
L	Last meal (time)
E	Events/environment

With the establishment of UK regional trauma centres, the UK trauma network is currently adopting the standardized ATMIST approach to delivering pre-hospital information to receiving hospitals.

MICRO-facts

ATMIST

A	Age
T	Time of incident
M	Mechanism of injury
I	Injuries
S	Signs and symptoms
T	Treatment delivered

12.2 COMPROMISED AIRWAY

Causes

- Decreased level of consciousness
- Neck trauma
- Facial trauma
- Severe burns
- Inhaled foreign body/vomitus/blood

Clinical features

- Cyanosis
- Stridor: Sign of upper airway obstruction
- Unconscious patient

Management

- Maintain airway with cervical spine triple immobilization:
  - Hard collar, sandbags and straps
  - Manual in-line cervical stabilization (MILS) during airway procedure
- High-flow oxygen via non-rebreathe mask
- Remove vomit/blood foreign bodies: suction with Yankauer sucker/McGills forceps under direct vision
- Airway adjunct:
  - Jaw thrust/chin lift: avoid head tilt to prevent further potential C-spine injury
  - Oropharyngeal airway: avoid nasopharyngeal in head injury (potential for basal skull fracture)
  - Formal intubation with cuffed oral endotracheal tube (COETT)
  - Surgical airway (needle/surgical cricothyroidectomy)

MICRO-reference

Follow ATLS protocol: Advanced Trauma Life Support for Doctors. *ATLS Student Course Manual*, 8th ed. American College of Surgeons Committee on Trauma, 2008.

Emergency and acute medicine

12.3 CERVICAL SPINE INJURY

Initial management

- Perform cervical spine immobilization if any of the following:
  - GCS <15 on initial assessment
  - Midline cervical pain or tenderness on palpation
  - Limb paraesthesia/focal neurology
  - Age >65 years old
  - Dangerous mechanism of injury
  - Any other clinical suspicion of cervical spine injury, especially with a concurrent painful distracting injury to torso or limbs
- Maintain immobilization until a full risk assessment, examination and any necessary imaging indicate it safe to remove. The patient should be able to comfortably rotate their neck to 45° or more bilaterally with an absence of developing neurological symptoms in order to clear the cervical spine clinically.
- The Canadian and Nexus C-spine rules may be used to aid this clinical decision-making process.

> **MICRO-reference**
> Head injury: NICE Guideline, http://guidance.nice.org.uk/CG56/ NICEGuidance/pdf/English

> **MICRO-reference**
> The Canadian C-Spine Rule, http://www.emottawa.ca/assets/ documents/research/cdr_cspine_poster.pdf

> **MICRO-reference**
> Nexus Criteria for C-Spine Imaging, http://www.mdcalc.com/ nexus-criteria-for-c-spine-imaging/

Investigations

- Plain radiograph of lateral cervical spine: viewing C1-C7/T1 interface (Fig. 12.2)
- Followed by AP and peg views
- CT C-spine should be performed if:
  - GCS below 13 on initial assessment
  - Has been intubated
  - Plain film series is technically inadequate (for example, desired view unavailable, suspicious or definitely abnormal)

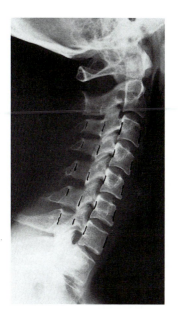

Fig. 12.2 Plain radiograph of cervical spine. (From Fig. 29.4b from Solomon, L. et al., *Apley's Concise System of Orthopaedics and Fractures*, 3rd edition, CRC Press, 2005.)

- Continued clinical suspicion of injury despite a normal X-ray
- The patient is being scanned for multi-region trauma

MICRO-reference
Cervical spine injury: NICE Guideline, http://guidance.nice.org.uk/ CG56/NICEGuidance/pdf/English

---

Management

- Immobilization:
  - Above and below suspected spinal injury
  - Semi-rigid cervical collar e.g. Philadelphia collar
  - Keep neck in neutral position
- Early intubation if respiratory compromise
- IV fluids to maintain normovolaemia
- Analgesia: see Section 1.3

MICRO-reference
Refer to ATLS guidelines: Advanced Trauma Life Support for Doctors. *ATLS Student Course Manual*, 8th ed. American College of Surgeons Committee on Trauma, 2008.

Emergency and acute medicine

12.4 BREATHING

Assessment
- Look:
  - Chest wall injury – bruising, deformity, wounds, flail chest
  - Accessory muscle use
  - Symmetrical chest movement
- Palpate:
  - Deviation of trachea
  - Percuss chest
- Auscultate:
  - Assess degree of air entry and quality of breathing

Investigations
- Regular observations:
  - Respiratory rate
  - Oxygen saturations
  - Blood pressure
  - Heart rate
- ABG: Hypoxia
- ECG
- Chest radiograph

Management
- Oxygen: Adjust according to oxygen saturations
- Assisted ventilation

12.5 CIRCULATION

If the patient has no pulse, refer to cardiac arrest guidelines (see Fig. 1.2).

12.6 TRAUMATIC HAEMORRHAGIC SHOCK

Definition
- Acute loss of blood or fluids
- Results in inadequate tissue perfusion
- Must be treated urgently
- Find precipitating cause and treat

Clinical features

- HR: ↑ HR drops pre-arrest
- BP: ↓
- Capillary refill time: ↓
- Urine output: ↓
- Decreased GCS

Management

- Aim to restore normal tissue perfusion
- Follow algorithm (Fig. 12.3)

> **MICRO-facts**
>
> New trauma guidelines also recommend the use of 1 g tranexamic acid in traumatic haemorrhagic shock.

DISABILITY

Definition

- Level of consciousness, i.e. assessing cerebral perfusion

Assessment

- Glasgow coma scale: see MICRO-facts
- Pupils: size, reaction
- Spinal injury:
    - Sensation
    - Power
    - Reflexes
- Do not forget glucose as a cause of fluctuating/reduced consciousness:
    - Check bedside blood glucose; monitor/serum glucose

Emergency and acute medicine

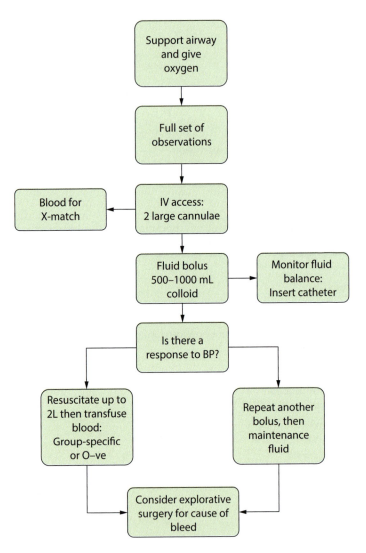

Fig. 12.3 Management of haemorrhagic shock.

MICRO-facts

Glasgow Coma Scale

EYES OPENING		MOTOR RESPONSE	
Spontaneously	4	On command	6
To voice	3	Localizes to pain	5
To pain	2	Flexes to pain	4
No response	1	Abnormal flexion	3
		Extends to pain	2
		No response	1

VERBAL RESPONSE	
Orientated	5
Confused	4
Inappropriate words	3
Incomprehensible sounds	2
No response	1

12.7 EXPOSURE

Definition
- To complete a full assessment by removal of patient's clothes as necessary

Management
- Adequate exposure to allow assessment of all injuries
- Perform thorough clinical examination
- Avoid hypothermia
- Try to maintain patient dignity at all times

12.8 POTENTIALLY LIFE-THREATENING INJURIES

TENSION PNEUMOTHORAX

Definition
- Progressive buildup of air within the pleural space that cannot return, creating a 'one-way valve' effect

- Increased pressure in the pleural space compresses the mediastinum to the opposite side, obstructing venous return to the heart
- Leads to circulatory failure and arrest if untreated

Aetiology

- Chest trauma:
  - Penetrating trauma:
    - Stabs
    - Gunshots
  - Blunt trauma

Clinical features

- Shocked unwell patient
- ↑ RR
- ↑ HR
- ↓ BP
- Hypoxic
- Distended neck veins
- Chest movements: asymmetrical and reduced
- Deviated trachea: away from affected side, as mediastinum is shifted to unaffected side
- Air entry: decreased or absent breath sounds on affected side
- Percussion: hyper-resonant on affected side
- Apex beat: displaces due to mediastinal shift

Management

- High-flow oxygen via face mask.
- Emergency chest decompression with a large-bore needle:
  - 14–16 G IV cannula.
  - Inserted into second rib space, midclavicular line (on side of pneumothorax).
- Insert an intercostal drain in the fifth intercostal space (ICS) just anterior to the mid-axillary line (triangle of safety) for the lung to expand and then remove the cannula from the second ICS on the same side.
- Request a plain chest radiograph after decompression and chest drain insertion.

TRAUMATIC PNEUMOTHORAX

Definition

- Chest trauma causing damage to the visceral or mediastinal pleura allowing air to enter the pleural space

Causes

- Blunt injury
- Penetrating
- Iatrogenic: insertion of chest drain

Clinical features

- Dependent on size of pneumothorax:
  - Shortness of breath
  - Pleuritic chest pain
  - ↑ RR
  - Cyanosis
  - ↓ Air entry: affected side
  - Hyper-resonance on percussion
  - Rib fractures: tenderness

Investigations

- Erect chest radiograph: free lung edge
- Oxygen saturations: reduced
- ABG: hypoxia

Management

- Oxygen: high flow (15 L)
- Analgesia
- Intercostal chest drain – do not insert through a chest wall wound
- May require mechanical ventilation

HAEMOTHORAX

Definition

- Collection of blood in the pleural space

Aetiology

- Blunt or penetrating injury:
  - Rib fractures
  - Lung parenchyma
  - Venous injury
  - Arterial injury

Clinical features

- ↑ RR
- Visible thoracic trauma: bruising, lacerations, penetrating injury
- Tenderness and crepitus on palpation: rib fracture
- Examine the back of chest also:
  - ↓ Chest movement
  - ↓ Air entry
  - Dull percussion note

Investigations

- Imaging: non-detectable injuries on exam
  - Plain chest radiograph: fluid level (massive haemothorax)
  - CT chest

- FAST ultrasound scan (focused assessment sonography in trauma) to identify free fluid (blood) in peritoneum or pericardium
  - Perihepatic
  - Perisplenic
  - Pelvis
  - Pericardium
- Withdrawal of blood through cannula to diagnose haemothorax

Management

- Drain blood via a large-bore intercostal chest drain inserted in the fifth ICS just anterior to the mid-axillary line.
- Thoracotomy if immediate drainage of 1000–1500 mL of blood (usually arterial injury) or >200 mL/h drainage for 2–4 h post-insertion of intercostal drain.

RIB FRACTURE

Aetiology

- Direct injury

Clinical features

- Sharp pain, exacerbated by inspiration, coughing, compression
- Tenderness and crepitus over ribs on palpation
- Respiratory and cardiac exam: exclude pneumothorax or other thoracic injuries

Management

- If uncomplicated, treating pain is sufficient: see Section 1.3
- Encourage breathing exercises
- Warn patient of delayed complications and to return if they develop severe chest pain and shortness of breath

FLAIL CHEST

Definition

- Multiple rib fractures can cause underlying lung damage (pulmonary contusions) and segments of chest wall to move independently

Clinical features

- Respiratory distress:
  - ↑ RR
  - Cyanosis
- Chest pain
- Paradoxical movement of flail segment: ineffective respiration
  - On inspiration: chest sucked inwards
  - On expiration: chest blown outwards

Investigations

- Oxygen saturations
- ABG:
  - Respiratory acidosis
  - Hypoxia
- Chest radiograph (Fig. 12.4):
  - Multiple rib fractures
  - Pneumothorax

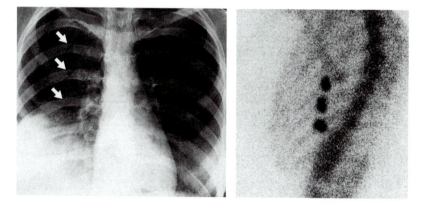

Fig. 12.4 Chest X-ray with multiple rib fractures. (From Fig. 29.15a from Solomon, L. et al., *Apley's Concise System of Orthopaedics and Fractures*, 3rd edition, CRC Press, 2005.)

Management

- Oxygen and ventilation: consider intermittent positive pressure ventilation (IPPV)
- Analgesia: see Section 1.3
- Often benefit from thoracic epidural or intercostal nerve block
- May need tracheal intubation if severe
- Treat associated injuries
- Discuss with cardiothoracic surgeons

CARDIAC TAMPONADE

Definition

- Accumulation of fluid in the pericardial space: pericardial effusion
- Pericardial pressure > ventricular filling pressure = reduced ventricular filling
- Untreated, will lead to cardiogenic shock: decreased cardiac output

Emergency and acute medicine

MICRO-print

Non-traumatic causes of cardiac tamponade

- Post-MI: Dressler syndrome
- Infections:
  - HIV
  - TB
  - Viral
- Connective tissue disease:
  - SLE
  - RA
- Latrogenic:
  - Pericardiocentesis
  - Pacemaker insertion
- Aortic dissection
- Cardiothoracic surgery
- Pericarditis
- Drugs
- Malignancy

Differential diagnosis

- Cardiogenic shock
- Tension pneumothorax

Clinical features

- Tachycardia/tachypnoea
- Dyspnoea
- Hypotension
- ↑ JVP/distended neck veins
- Pericardial rub
- Diminished heart sounds

Investigations

- See Table 12.1

Management

- Transfer to ICU
- Oxygen
- Fluid
- Medical:
  - Oxygen
  - Fluid resuscitation to maintain intravascular volume
  - Bed rest with leg elevation: increase venous return
  - Treat underlying cause to prevent recurrence

Table 12.1 **Initial investigations for cardiac tamponade**

INVESTIGATION	FINDING
ECG	• Sinus tachycardia
Chest radiograph	• Cardiomegaly • Bottle-shaped heart
Echocardiogram	• Compression • Reduced ventricular filling
Blood tests	• CK and troponin: raised in MI, trauma • Clotting profile: bleeding risk if intervention performed

- Surgical:
  - Urgent call to cardiothoracic team
  - Pericardiocentesis: removal of pericardial fluid
  - Open thoracotomy and/or pericardotomy
  - Pericardectomy
  - Pericardio-peritoneal shunt

AORTIC RUPTURE

> ### MICRO-facts
>
> The vast majority of these patients do not survive. The small proportion that do have multiple severe chest injuries, and therefore have a high index of suspicion for aortic rupture.

Mechanism of injury

- Shearing force
- Rapid deceleration
- Direct injury

Causes

- High-energy blunt trauma:
  - Major road traffic accidents
  - Falls from significant height
- Penetrating injury:
  - Stab or gunshot wounds

Clinical features

- Hypovolaemic shock
- Chest pain
- Back pain 'tearing'

Emergency and acute medicine

- Absent/weak or asymmetrical pulses
- BP difference between right and left arm or between arms and arms and legs

Investigations

- Ideally erect CXR if possible, but often only AP supine as part of a trauma series:
  - May be normal
  - Widened mediastinum (>8 cm at level of aortic arch)
  - Loss of aortic knuckle contour (easier to see if calcified)
  - Depression of left main stem bronchus
  - Apical cap (pleural haematoma)
  - Deviation of NGT (if present) to the right

Management

- High-flow oxygen
- IV access: two large-bore cannulae (14 G)
  - Take blood for cross-match: 6–8 units
  - Fluid resuscitation: colloid, up to 2 L if profoundly shocked. Allow permissive hypotension to prevent further bleeding until definitive treatment
- Regular monitoring of vital signs to measure effect of fluid on systemic filling:
  - Urinary catheter
  - Central line with CVP monitoring
  - Invasive BP monitoring via arterial line
- After 2 L fluid, consider blood transfusion: see Section 9.7
  - Group-specific blood
  - O negative blood
- Urgent CT aortic angiogram
- Urgent referral to vascular surgeons for repair: open repair or endovascular

ABDOMINAL INJURY

Causes

- Blunt injury:
  - Road accident
  - Crush injuries
  - Direct punch/kick
- Penetrating injury:
  - Knife wound
  - Gunshot

Affected organs

- Spleen: most commonly injured organ
- Liver: second most common but higher mortality due to difficulty controlling bleeding
- Kidneys: blunt injuries
- Bladder: consider further pelvic injury:
    - Pelvic haematoma
    - Fractured pelvis
    - Rectal
    - Vaginal
    - Bowel perforation
- Pancreas: rarely isolated trauma, usually part of multi-organ damage
- Abdominal aortic rupture: see above

Investigations

- Bloods:
    - FBC: Hb may be low or normal in acute blood loss
    - U&E: assess renal function
    - LFTs: assess for hepatic injury (raised transaminases)
    - Amylase: assess for pancreatic injury (raised)
    - Clotting screen: to assess risk of bleeding and may indicate hepatic impairment if deranged
    - Cross-match
- Urinalysis: look for blood and protein to assess for renal tract injury
- Erect CXR if possible: pneumoperitoneum (indicates perforation of viscus)
- AXR
- FAST (USS): haemoperitoneum and free intra-abdominal fluid (see MICRO-fact)
- Abdominal CT scan: identify affected organ and bleeding

MICRO-facts

FAST scan

Looks for free fluid in:
- Perihepatic (Morrison pouch)
- Perisplenic
- Pericardium
- Pelvis

Management

- Emergency explorative laparotomy if unstable
- Conservative management may be successful – 'watchful waiting'
- Pelvic stabilization

> **MICRO-facts**
>
> Pelvic fractures can be life threatening due to massive blood loss; in particular anterior-posterior or 'open book' fractures that increase pelvic volume can be difficult to control.

PELVIC FRACTURE

Causes

- Low-energy injuries: falls in the elderly
- High-energy injuries: fall from great height, road traffic collisions, crush injuries, ejection from motor vehicle

Examination

- See Table 12.2

Table 12.2 **Examination areas in pelvic fractures**

EXAM	FEATURES
Pelvic area	• Tenderness • Bleeding • Perineal or scrotal haematoma • Blood at urethral meatus • Open or closed fractures
Legs	• Leg length discrepancy • Asymmetrical rotation of hip
Rectum	• Prostate: position and mobility • Fractures • Blood in stool
Vaginal	• Palpable fractures • Size and consistency of uterus • Bleeding • Viable pregnancy

Investigations

- If a pelvic fracture is suspected, apply a pelvic binder to reduce the pelvic volume (thereby reducing bleeding) until radiographic imaging performed. Remove only once a fracture is excluded.

- Do not try to determine the stability of the pelvis by gentle compression – this should only be performed once, ideally by a senior orthopaedic surgeon.
- Bloods: baseline bloods prior to theatre:
  - FBC: Hb may be low or normal in acute blood loss.
  - U&E: assess renal function.
  - Clotting: to assess risk of bleeding/DIC/DVT.
  - Cross-match 6 units (for theatre).
- Imaging:
  - Pelvic radiograph: AP view (Fig. 12.5)
  - CT
  - Always exclude concurrent abdominal injury

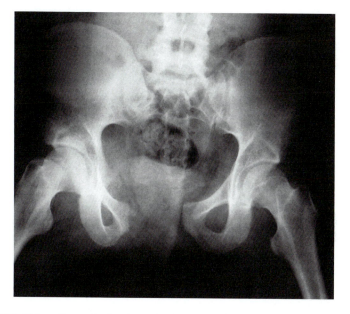

Fig. 12.5 Plain radiograph of an 'open book' injury pelvic fracture. (From Solomon, L. et al., *Apley's Concise System of Orthopaedics and Fractures*, 3rd edition, CRC Press, Boca Raton, FL, 2005, Fig. 30.6a.)

MICRO-facts

The bony pelvis is a ring that rarely sustains an isolated injury. Always look for more than one fracture.

Management

- Do not attempt repeated manipulation of a fractured pelvis: there is a risk of massive haemorrhage
- Resuscitation with IV fluids
- Insert urinary catheter: if no contraindications
  - Urethral injury
  - Abnormal 'high riding' prostate on rectal exam
- Call orthopaedics to review urgently for surgical fixation
- May also need interventional radiology for coiling of bleeding pelvic vessels
- Symptomatic treatment: strong analgesia; see Section 1.3

HEAD INJURY

Definition

- Trauma to the head, other than superficial injuries to the face

Causes

- Direct blow to head:
  - Contusions
  - Laceration
  - Penetrating injury
  - Intracranial bleed
  - Fractures
  - Raised intracranial pressure
- Hypoxia

Clinical features

- Headache
- Loss of consciousness
- Amnesia
- Vomiting
- Periorbital haematoma: 'raccoon eyes' (Fig. 12.6)
- Focal neurology
- Leakage of CSF and/or blood from nose or ears
- Mastoid bruising
- Haematoma
- Seizures
- Haemotympanum

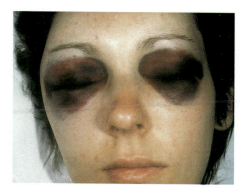

Fig. 12.6 Periorbital haematoma. (From Solomon, L. et al., *Apley's Concise System of Orthopaedics and Fractures*, 3rd edition, CRC Press, Boca Raton, FL, 2005, Fig. 22.5.)

MICRO-facts

Remember to look behind the ears on inspection. 'Battle sign' is bruising behind the mastoid process and indicates a basal skull fracture.

Investigations

- CT head (Fig. 12.7)
- Skull X-rays are no longer routinely performed

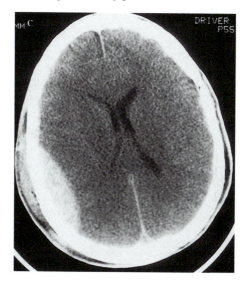

Fig. 12.7 CT scan of an extradural haematoma following a head injury. (From Solomon, L. et al., *Apley's Concise System of Orthopaedics and Fractures*, 3rd edition, CRC Press, Boca Raton, FL, 2005, Fig. 22.6c.)

Emergency and acute medicine

> ## MICRO-facts
>
> ### Criteria for CT head
> Any one of the following:
> - GCS <13 on initial assessment
> - GCS <15 two hours after initial assessment
> - Sign of open or depressed fracture at skull base
> - Post-traumatic seizure
> - Focal neurology
> - >1 episode vomiting
> - Amnesia >30 min
> - Loss of consciousness plus age >65, coagulopathy and/or patient on warfarin, 'dangerous mechanism of injury'
> - Persistent complaint related to head injury <48 h of discharge

Management

- See Fig. 12.8
- Admit the patient for further investigation and treatment if:
  - Difficult to assess:
    - Post-ictal
    - Drug/alcohol intoxication
    - Multiple injuries
  - GCS <15 after imaging
  - Continual worrying signs:
    - Severe headache
    - Persistent vomiting
- Regular observations:
  - Neuro observation (GCS, pupils, peripheral neurology, vital observations) every 30 min until GCS is 15/15, then hourly for 4 h, then 4 hourly
- Assess amnesia
- Do not discharge patients until GCS is 15/15 and symptoms well controlled
- Give verbal and written advice on head injury and advise a sober friend/relative to accompany patient home and observe closely for 24 h
- Alert patient on the possibility of delayed complications
- Arrange GP follow-up for those who have undergone CT head or have been admitted

> ### MICRO-reference
> Head injury: NICE Guideline, http://guidance.nice.org.uk/CG56/NICEGuidance/pdf/English

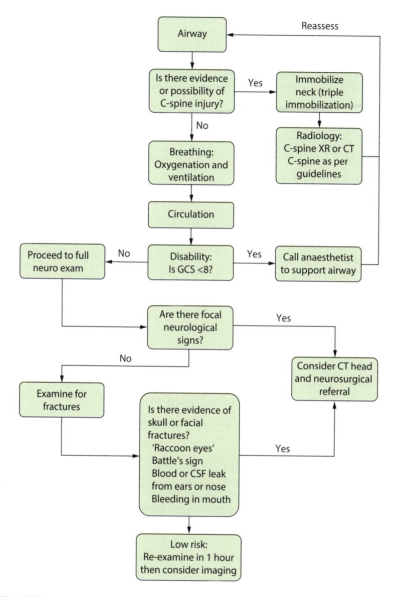

Fig. 12.8 Immediate management of head injury.

MICRO-facts

Do not discharge any patient who presents with a head injury until GCS is 15/15 and any symptoms are well controlled.

Complications
- Deterioration of GCS
- Extradural/subdural haematoma
- Seizures
- Permanent neurological deficit
- Diabetes insipidus

FACIAL INJURY

Definition
- Any injury to the face:
  - Soft tissue injury:
    - Burns
    - Lacerations
    - Bruises
  - Fractures:
    - Facial
    - Nasal
    - Jaw
  - Eye injury – globe/lens/retinal injuries/corneal abrasions

MICRO-facts

Head, chest and abdominal trauma take precedence over facial injuries; however, until proven otherwise, the airway is threatened and therefore airway compromise should be excluded first.

Aetiology
- Assault:
  - Domestic violence
  - Alcohol
- Road traffic accident
- Falls
- Sport injuries

Associated injuries
- Head injury
- Cervical spine injury

> **MICRO-facts**
>
> All maxillofacial and head injuries have presumed concurrent cervical spine injury until proven otherwise.

Clinical features

- See Table 12.3
- Pain
- Swelling
- Asymmetry
- Bleeding
- Numbness
- Crepitus

Table 12.3 **Assessment of facial injuries**

HISTORY	EXAMINATION
Cause	• Facial asymmetry • Lacerations/abrasions
Degree of force	• Palpable deformities • Fractured bones or teeth
Specific symptoms	• Visual disturbances: diplopia, reflexes, visual acuity, visual fields, papillary responses and corneal abrasions (use fluorescein and a slit lamp)
Time since injury	• Intranasal inspection for nasal septal haematoma, which requires urgent drainage under ENT to prevent septal necrosis
Systemic history	• Facial movement • Facial sensation

Investigations

- CT head: in case of associated head injury (haematoma)
- Cervical spine radiograph: associated cervical spine injury until proven otherwise (fractures)

Management

- ABC resuscitation:
  - Is the airway at risk?
  - Is breathing impaired?
  - Control any bleeding
- Pain control: see Section 1.3
- Open wounds: suture/bandage
- Swelling: ice

- Antibiotic cover
- Check tetanus status: consider booster cover
- C-spine and/or head injury: see cervical spine injury/head injury section
- Jaw dislocations:
  - Analgesia/sedation
  - Reduce

Complications

- Airway compromise
- Aspiration
- Bleeding
- Infection
- Alert patient to potential future complications:
  - Scars
  - Facial deformity (can lead to psychosocial problems)
  - Nerve damage: altered sense of smell, taste, vision, sensation
  - Delayed union or non-union
- Chronic breathing problems

MAXILLOFACIAL FRACTURES

Nasal fracture

Aetiology

- Lateral or anterior direct blow:
  - Punch
  - Direct fall

Clinical features

- Pain
- Swelling/deformity
- Epistaxis
- Lacerations
- Respiratory obstruction

Investigations

- Clinical diagnosis
- Facial X-ray or CT head: if other fractures or head injury suspected

Management

- Clean wounds
- Analgesia: see Section 1.3
- Antibiotic course if open wound and punch injury e.g. co-amoxiclav or amoxicillin
- Pack with nasal tampon or nasal balloon device if ongoing epistaxis despite nose pinching for 30 min/ice

- Refer to ENT:
  - Septal haematoma. Will need incision and drainage to prevent septal necrosis and needs antibiotic cover.
  - Significantly deviated nose. Others can be followed up at 10 days in an ENT outpatient clinic.
  - Significant bleeding requiring nasal packing
- Treat associated head injury (see 'Head injury')

Zygomatic (malar) fracture

Aetiology

- Direct blunt trauma to face

Clinical features

- Pain
- Swelling
- Numbness to cheek
- Associated eye injuries: Lid swelling
- Haematoma
- Depression at fracture site
- Surgical emphysema/crepitus

Investigations

- Facial plain radiograph
- Cervical spine plain radiograph
- CT facial bones

Management

- Patient should not blow their nose
- Refer to maxillofacial surgery and ophthalmology for treatment

Maxillary fracture

Aetiology

- High-energy injury

Grading

- Le Fort classification; see Table 12.4

Table 12.4 **Classification of maxillary fractures using the Le Fort classification**

LE FORT CLASSIFICATION	FRACTURE LINE	AFFECTED FEATURES
Le Fort I	Transmaxillary	• Teeth • Soft palate • Hard palate

(Continued)

Table 12.4 *(Continued)* **Classification of maxillary fractures using the Le Fort classification**

LE FORT CLASSIFICATION	FRACTURE LINE	AFFECTED FEATURES
Le Fort II	Pyramidal/ subzygomatic	• Nasal bones • Maxilla • Lower orbits
Le Fort III	Craniofacial	• Maxilla • Nasal bones • Base of skull

Clinical features

- Swelling: facial
- Bleeding:
  - Facial
  - Pharyngeal: may lead to airway obstruction
- Bruising:
  - Facial
  - Periorbital: raccoon eyes
- Facial deformity: lengthening
- CSF rhinorrhoea
- Mobile and tender bones
- Mobile hard palate
- Misaligned teeth

Management

- Establish patent airway and resuscitate. The fractured face may need to be pulled forwards by applying traction to the upper jaw.
- Control bleeding with packing/facial traction.
- Clean small facial wounds and cover with steristrips.
- Prophylactic antibiotics: co-amoxiclav or amoxicillin.
- Refer to maxillofacial team for reduction and fixation of fractures.
- Neurosurgery referral if basal skull fracture/intracranial injury.

Orbital fracture

Aetiology

- Direct blow to eye:
  - Rapid compression of tissues
  - ↑ Intraorbital pressure

> **MICRO-facts**
>
> Perform a full eye examination including use of fundoscope, Snellen chart, slit lamp.

Clinical features

- Pain
- Swelling
- Ecchymoses of eyelids
- Subconjunctival haemorrhage
- Facial asymmetry
- Facial numbness
- Enopthalmos (eyeball recession)
- Visual disturbance:
    - Diplopia
    - Blindness
- May be visible eye injury:
    - Retinal detachment
    - Glaucoma
    - Surgical emphysema
- Test function of nerves
- Abnormal eye movements if inferior rectus trapped in orbital floor fracture
- Visual acuity

Investigations

- CT scan: if neurological symptoms/associated head injury
- X-rays do not always identify orbital floor fractures

Management

- Urgent ophthalmology referral for orbital decompression

Mandibular fracture
Aetiology

- Intraoral injury
- Direct blow to jaw
- Head injury

Clinical features

- Pain: on biting
- Malocclusion or loose teeth
- Excessive salivation
- Dysphagia
- Swelling
- Crepitation
- Deformity

Investigations

- Orthopantomogram (OPT):
    - Multiple fractures

- Mandibular dislocation – diagnosed clinically. Simple dislocation does not require X-ray and should be reduced by downward pressure on the lower molars bilaterally using both thumbs (well padded with gauze to prevent injury from the patient biting down during the reduction).

Management

- Simple fracture:
  - Analgesia: see Section 1.3
  - Prophylactic antibiotics, e.g. co-amoxiclav 500 mg TDS or amoxicillin 500 mg
  - Assess tetanus status: consider booster
  - Arrange follow-up with maxillofacial surgeons
- Multiple fractures or dislocation:
  - Refer to maxillofacial surgeons for reduction and further investigation

12.9 BITES

Aetiology

- Always check and document tetanus status
- Animal: bites are infected until proven otherwise: give prophylactic antibiotics
- Human: caused during fights: common infective organisms: staphylococci, streptococci, anaerobes

Investigations

- Obtain radiograph of bitten limb: foreign bodies, fractures
- Swab wound for culture and sensitivity

Management

- Clean wound: may need debridement and wash out
- Remove foreign bodies
- Dress and splint wound
- Bites should generally not be sutured due to infection risk and may require secondary closure at 3–5 days
- Give prophylactic antibiotics: co-amoxiclav 625 mg TDS 7 days

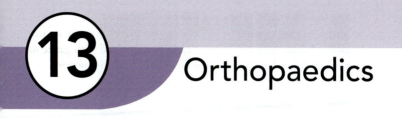

13 Orthopaedics

13.1 FRACTURES

Definition
- Disruption in all or part of the cortex of the bone

Describing a fracture
- See Table 13.1

Table 13.1 **Describing a fracture**

KEY POINTS TO COVER	DETAILS
Location of fracture	• Side: dominant or non-dominant (upper limb) • Site • Section of bone
Direction of fracture related to long axis of the bone	• Transverse/perpendicular • Diagonal/oblique: same direction as axis • Longitudinal: along long axis • Spiral: twisting fracture along bone
Position: relationship of distal fragment relative to proximal fragment	• Displacement • Angulation • Shortening/impaction: overlapping of fragments • Rotation
Number of fracture segments	• Simple: 2 fragments • Comminuted: >2
Distal neurovascular state	• Pulses • Doppler signals • Capillary refill • Neurological deficit – sensory and motor
Communication with external environment	• Open (compound) • Closed

Investigations
- Plain radiograph of affected limb: two views (antero-posterior [AP] and lateral) (Fig. 13.1)

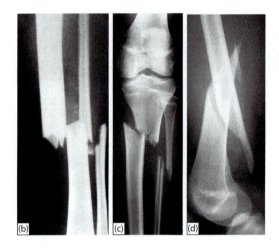

Fig. 13.1 X-rays of different fractures. (From Solomon, L. et al., *Apley's Concise System of Orthopaedics and Fractures*, 3rd edition, CRC Press, Boca Raton, FL, 2005, Fig 23.1b–d.)

Management

- General principles:
  - Analgesia
  - Thorough examination
  - Immobilization
  - Orthopaedic review
  - Advice:
    - Simple fractures heal over 6 weeks
    - More complicated/severe fractures may decrease range of movement permanently

13.2 OPEN FRACTURE

Definition

- Communication between external environment and bone

Clinical features

- History: mechanism of injury (where, how did it occur?)
- Examination: appropriate joint examination, assess neurovascular status

Investigations

- Plain radiograph of fracture:
  - Two views
  - Usually AP and lateral
- Tetanus status: consider booster/immunoglobulin

- Bloods:
  - FBC
  - U&E
  - Group and save (preparation for surgery)
  - Consider cross-match if there is profuse bleeding or risk of blood loss in theatre

Management

- Analgesia
- Debridement and lavage
- Dressing
- Reduce and splint fracture
- Antibiotics: e.g. co-amoxiclav 1.2 g TDS or cefuroxime 1.5 g TDS; consider a stat dose of gentamicin 1.5 mg/kg at time of surgery
- Keep nil by mouth (NBM)
- Refer to orthopaedics (patient will need to go to theatre for aggressive debridement and stabilization of fracture)

13.3 UPPER LIMB FRACTURES

- See Figs. 13.2 through 13.4 for examples of Colles' fracture, scaphoid fracture, and Smith's fracture, respectively.
- See Table 13.2 for information regarding upper limb fractures.

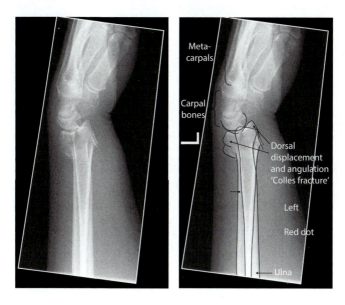

Fig. 13.2 Colles' fracture. (From Walker, A. et al., *Clinical Investigations on the Move*, CRC Press, Boca Raton, FL, 2012, Fig. 5.21.)

Emergency and acute medicine

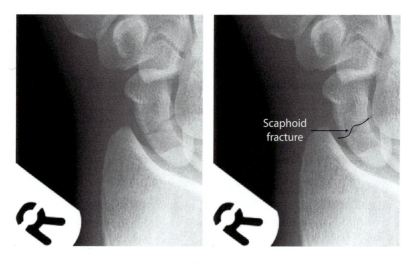

Fig. 13.3 Scaphoid fracture. (From Walker, A. et al., *Clinical Investigations on the Move*, CRC Press, Boca Raton, FL, 2012, Fig. 5.23.)

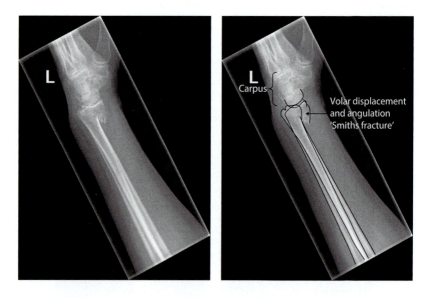

Fig. 13.4 Smith's fracture. (From Walker, A. et al., *Clinical Investigations on the Move*, CRC Press, Boca Raton, FL, 2012, Fig. 5.22.)

Emergency and acute medicine

Table 13.2 Upper limb fractures: mechanism of injury, clinical features and management

MECHANISM OF INJURY	FRACTURE	CLINICAL FEATURES	MANAGEMENT

Fall onto outstretched hand	• Colles' fracture:
	  • Distal radius ± ulnar styloid
	  • Distal bony segment displaced dorsally
		• 'Dinner fork' deformity
		• Wrist tenderness
		• Check neurovascular status
			• Analgesia
			• Immobilize in plaster of paris
			• Elevate: high arm sling
			• Encourage movement
			• Fracture clinic:
			  • Consider manipulation or reduction with orthopaedics (if displaced)

Fall onto dorsum of hand (flexed wrist)	• Smith's fracture:
	  • Volar displacement of distal radius
	  • Reverse Colles' fracture
	  • Unstable fracture
		• 'Garden spade' deformity
		• Pain and tenderness
			• Analgesia
			• Immobilize in plaster of paris
			• Refer to orthopaedics
			• Manipulation under anaesthetic or open reduction with internal fixation

Punch injury	• Fractured fifth metacarpal bone	• Rotational deformity: overlapping of fingers on flexion into palm	• Neighbour 'buddy' strapping or ulnar gutter for more displaced fractures requiring manipulation
			• Elevate: high arm sling
			• Analgesia
			• Encourage hand exercises
			• Treat for any bites:
			  • Broad-spectrum antibiotics
			  • Tetanus status

(Continued)

Emergency and acute medicine

Table 13.2 (Continued) Upper limb fractures: mechanism of injury, clinical features and management

MECHANISM OF INJURY	FRACTURE	CLINICAL FEATURES	MANAGEMENT

Direct trauma to wrist
Fall onto outstretched hand
	• Scaphoid fracture	• Tender over anatomical snuffbox
		• Pain and swelling in radial aspect of wrist over scaphoid tubercle and on thumb telescoping
		• Poor grip
			• Analgesia
			• Futura wrist splint or plaster of paris
			• Review in 10–14 days with follow-up X-ray (not always visible initially)
			• Complication: avascular necrosis:
			  • Suspect if persistent pain/tenderness at follow-up
			  • Requires bone scan if follow-up X-ray normal and still clinical suspicion of fracture

Direct trauma to elbow Fall onto outstretched wrist	• Radial head/neck fracture	• Elbow effusion • Inability to fully extend and flex elbow • Tenderness over radial head on palpation pronation/supination	• Analgesia • Collar and cuff • Immobilize in plaster of paris if displaced and elevate in high arm sling • Fracture clinic • May need sedation and manipulation or internal fixation if displaced
Direct trauma Fall onto outstretched hand Fall onto shoulder	• Clavicle fracture	• Tenderness over clavicle • Check neurovascular state and overlying skin for tenting/wounds • Examine for associated spinal injuries	• Analgesia • Broad arm sling • Fracture clinic (rarely need fixation)

13.4 LOWER LIMB FRACTURES

HIP FRACTURE

Definition
- Fractured neck of femur (see Fig. 13.5)
- Intracapsular
- Extracapsular

Clinical features
- Pain, exacerbated by:
  - Weight bearing
  - Movement of affected hip; flexion, extension, internal and external rotation

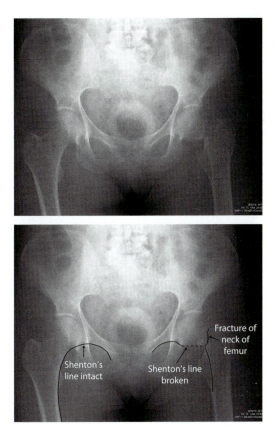

Fig. 13.5 X-ray showing a neck of femur fracture. (From Fig. 5.20 from NOF#-CR0001-edited.TIF [Google docs].)

- Patients may complain of knee pain (referred to as pain via obturator nerve)
- Affected leg appears shorter and externally rotated

Investigations

- Bloods:
  - FBC: baseline Hb in case blood transfusion is necessary
  - U&E: assess renal function (many elderly patients are dehydrated)
  - Glucose: to exclude cause of fall if unknown (hypoglycaemia)
  - Clotting profile: to assess bleeding risk and in preparation for theatre
  - Group and save
  - Cross-match 2 units (prepare patient for theatre)
- ECG: look for cause of fall if unknown or in elderly patient (arrhythmia, MI)
- Plain radiograph of hip (anterior-posterior and lateral)
- CXR: to assess suitability for theatre and treat any underlying medical problems (such as a concurrent chest infection)

MICRO-facts

It is vital to rule out intracapsular fractures, which can compromise the blood supply to the femoral head leading to avascular necrosis.

Management

- Venous thromboembolic prophylaxis: See Chapter 9, Haematology
- IV fluids
- Strong IV analgesia: see Section 1.3 or fascia-iliaca nerve block
- Antiemetic e.g. metoclopramide 10 mg, max. 8 hourly
- Refer to orthopaedics for repair
- Manage comorbidities in elderly patients
- If the surgery is likely to be delayed until the next day then repeat Hb in the morning

FEMORAL SHAFT FRACTURE

Aetiology

- High-energy trauma:
  - Fall from height
  - Crush injuries
  - Severe road traffic accident

Clinical features

- Deformity: shortening and external rotation
- Pain
- Swelling/haematoma (up to 1 L of blood); may have profuse bleeding if open fracture
- Multiple injuries:
  - Examine for associated hip, pelvic, lower limb and spinal injuries
  - Full neurovascular exam
  - Head injury (GCS)
- Complications:
  - Hypovolaemic shock (severe blood loss)
  - Cardiogenic shock (chest injuries: pneumothorax)
  - Compartment syndrome

Investigations

- Plain radiograph of hip and full length femur: two views (anterior-posterior and lateral)

Management

- ABC: resuscitation
- IV access: give fluids and take blood (cross-match for theatre)
- Appropriate analgesia: opioid and femoral nerve block/three-in-one block if more proximal
- Immobilize in Thomas splint, then order plain radiograph of femur
- Refer to orthopaedics for repair (commonly intramedullary nail)

ANKLE FRACTURE

Clinical features

- Unable to weight-bear immediately after injury
- Painful, swollen, tender ankle joint with painfully restricted ROM

Investigations

- Plain radiograph of ankle according to Ottawa ankle rules (see MICRO-print)
- Talar shift (gap between medial mallelous and talus) requires orthopaedic intervention
- Fractured bone may be visible
- If there is a high clinical suspicion of fracture dislocation, reduce immediately under sedation/analgesia prior to radiology to prevent neurovascular compromise

> **MICRO-print**
>
> **Ottawa ankle rules**
>
> When to use radiography to view injuries to the ankle:
> - Unable to weight bear immediately following injury or in the ED
> - Tenderness over distal 6 cm posterior surface or tip of lateral or medial malleolus
> - X-ray of foot in addition if fifth MT base or navicular tenderness
>
> Following these rules results in a low rate of false negatives on imaging.

Management

- Rest
- Elevation
- Ice
- Analgesia: see Section 1.3
- Small fractures (may be treated as sprain): early mobilization/ankle support compression bandage
- Larger fractures: immobilization/NWB and orthopaedic referral
- May require open reduction and internal fixation

13.5 FRACTURE COMPLICATIONS

- See Table 13.3

Table 13.3 **Complications of a fracture**

COMPLICATIONS OF A FRACTURE	LOCAL	GENERAL
Immediate	• Open fracture • Skin loss or compromise • Nerve palsy • Vascular injury: ischaemia	• Bleeding • Hypovolaemic shock
Early	• Compartment syndrome • Infection	• DVT • Fat embolus
Late	• Delayed union and non-union • Joint stiffness • Chronic osteomyelitis	• Poor mobility

COMPARTMENT SYNDROME

Definition
- Increased pressure in a muscle compartment due to bleeding, oedema or infection leading to reduced blood flow and further increased pressure and ischaemia

Causes
- Fracture
- Crush injuries to soft tissues
- Tight cast

Clinical features
- Most common:
  - Lower leg (tibial fractures)
  - Forearm
- Less common:
  - Hand
  - Foot
  - Upper arm
- Pain disproportionate to clinical context
- ↓ Limb sensation
- Tightening sensation across skin
- Muscle compartment feels firm
- Skin discoloration
- Weakness
- Swelling

MICRO-facts

Compartment syndrome
If sensation is lost and peripheral pulses non-palpable then the limb is immediately threatened and this is a surgical emergency.

Investigations
- Measure compartment pressures in affected leg
- Doppler device: measure presence and quality of pulses

Management
- Open fasciotomy: urgent decompression

Complications
- Permanent damage to nerves
- Loss of function to affected limb

- May occur up to 12–24 h following compression
- Volkmann's ischaemic contracture:
  - Ischaemic injury to muscles of forearm
  - Muscle replaced by fibrous tissue leading to deformity
  - Can occur following:
    - Fractures
    - Crush injuries
    - Compartment syndrome
- Amputation may be needed if the limb cannot be saved
  - Consider palliative care

COMMON NERVE INJURIES

- See Table 13.4

Table 13.4 **Common nerve injuries**

NERVE	CAUSES	MOTOR LOSS	SENSORY LOSS
Axilliary	• Shoulder dislocation • Humeral head fracture	• Shoulder abduction, weak flexion, extension and rotation of the shoulder	• Lateral aspect of shoulder • 'Regimental badge' area
Median	• Supracondylar fractures of humerus • Lacerations at wrist	• Weak pronation of forearm • Unable to adduct thumb against resistance	• Radial/lateral 3½ fingers (including thumb) • Corresponding area of palm
Ulnar	• Elbow compression • Fracture at medial epicondyle • Wrist injury	• Little finger • Abduction/adduction • 'Clawing'	• Palmar • Medial 1½ fingers
Radial	• Humeral shaft fracture • Compression in axilla	• Inability to extend wrist; 'wrist drop'	• Dorsum first web space
Common peroneal	• Knee dislocation • Tibial fracture	• Inability to dorsiflex foot • 'Foot drop'	• Numbness in lateral lower leg and foot

13.6 OSTEOPOROTIC FRACTURES

Definition
- Usually low-energy injuries

Fracture sites

Table 13.5 **Common sites of osteoporotic fractures**

FRACTURE SITES	FRACTURE	CLINICAL FEATURES
Spine	• Vertebral wedge compression fracture	• Thoracic back pain • Follows minor injury • Loss in height • Kyphotic spine deformity
Wrist	• Colles' fracture	• (See upper limb fractures)
Hip	• Neck of femur fracture	• (See hip fractures)

Management
- Analgesia: see Section 1.3
- Early mobilization/physiotherapy
- Refer to GP for treatment of underlying osteoporosis:
  - Calcium supplements
  - Vitamin D
  - Bisphosphonates
- Consider bone densitometry scan (DEXA)

13.7 DISLOCATIONS

Definition
- There is complete disruption of the joint
- The bony articular components of the joint are no longer in contact with each other

SHOULDER

Types
- Anterior: forced abduction/external rotation
- Posterior: less common (see Fig. 13.6)

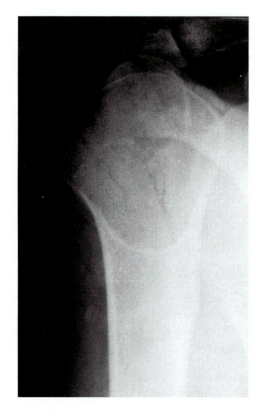

Fig. 13.6 Plain radiograph of posterior shoulder dislocation. (From Solomon, L. et al., *Apley's Concise System of Orthopaedics and Fractures*, 3rd edition, CRC Press, Boca Raton, FL, 2005, Fig. 26.8.)

Aetiology

- Seizures
- Electrocution
- Fall onto internally rotated arm

Clinical features

- Severe pain
- Difficulty moving arm (often patient is supporting with good arm)
- Bulge under clavicle
- Gap below acromion
- Loss of shoulder contour
- Shoulder examination:
  - Confirm neurovascular status of upper limb:
    - Distal pulses
    - Sensation in region of axillary nerve (regimental badge)

Investigations

- Plain radiograph of shoulder (two views):
  - Anterior:
    - Humeral head lies anterior and inferior to glenoid
  - Posterior:
    - 'Light bulb' sign
    - Abnormal symmetry between humeral head and glenoid

Management

- Analgesia: sedation or Entonox
- Relocate by manipulation:
  - Modified Milch technique
  - Kocher's method
- Collar and cuff sling to hold in place post-reduction
- Repeat plain radiograph of shoulder to ensure full reduction
- Re-examine pulses and sensation
- Arrange follow-up with orthopaedics and physiotherapy
- Explain the increased risk of dislocation in the future
- Discharge patient with analgesia

ANKLE

> ## MICRO-facts
> This is an orthopaedic emergency!

Clinical features

- Gross deformity of ankle
- May be associated with open fractures
- Severe skin tension
- Neurological deficit: decreased sensation and pulses

Investigations

- Urgent reduction should be performed before radiographic imaging
- Photograph and document any open wounds before irrigating well with sterile saline and dressing

Management

- Immediate senior help
- Sedation: Entonox or strong IV analgesia
- Urgent reduction and immobilization in plaster avoiding equinas positioning of the foot
- Re-examine for distal sensation and pulses
- Urgent referral to orthopaedics

Emergency and acute medicine

SOFT TISSUE INJURY

Definition

- Damage to muscles, tendons or ligaments

Aetiology

- Tearing or overstretching of ligaments/muscle/tendon
- Ligaments get sprained
- Muscles get strained

Clinical features

- Pain
- Tenderness
- Soft tissue swelling

Management

- Rest: initially, then weight-bear when symptoms improve
- Ice: reduce swelling
- Compression
- Elevation: reduce swelling and pain
- Analgesia: paracetamol and ibuprofen (see Section 1.3)
- Minor sprain: reassure and encourage early mobilization as symptoms allow
- Physiotherapy
- Ruptured ligament or extreme laxity of joint: refer for surgery

13.8 KNEE INJURIES

Ottawa knee rules can be used to decide whether radiographic imaging is required or not:

- Inability to weight bear immediately at time of injury or unable to take four steps in the ED
- Fibular head tenderness
- Inability to flex knee to 90°
- Age >55 years old
- Isolated patella tenderness

MICRO-facts

Referred hip pain can present with knee pain alone; therefore it is important to examine both hip and knee.

RUPTURED ANTERIOR CRUCIATE LIGAMENT

Aetiology
- Sports injury: particularly rugby, football and skiing

Clinical features
- 'Popping' sound
- Unable to weight-bear
- Immediate swelling
- Pain on flexion
- Unstable knee: feeling of 'giving way'
- Decreased range of movement
- Positive anterior draw test
- Positive Lachmann test
- Positive bulge test: effusion

Investigations
- Plain radiograph of knee (AP and lateral views): may be normal
- MRI knee

Management
- Conservative:
  - Rest
  - Ice
  - Elevation
- Knee support: splint and non-weight bearing with crutches
- Physiotherapy: strengthen surrounding muscles and stabilize joint
- Surgical: reconstruction of ACL

MENISCAL TEAR

Clinical features
- History of twisting injury to knee: football, rugby
- Pain: relieved by rest
- Swelling
- Effusion
- Joint line tenderness
- 'Locked knee' (unable to fully extend knee)
- McMurray test positive

Investigations
- Plain radiograph: normal
- MRI: reliable for identifying tears

Emergency and acute medicine

Management

- Analgesia
- Knee support
- Physiotherapy
- Arthroscopic surgery: investigate and repair; required urgently if evidence of locked knee

13.9 ACUTE BACK PAIN

Aetiology

- Traumatic injury
- Leaking aortic aneurysm
- Cord compression
- Cauda equina syndrome (posterior disc prolapse)
- Mechanical back pain
- Infection: abscess/discitis
- Vertebral collapse fracture
- Spondylitis
- Renal colic
- Malignancy e.g. multiple myeloma

Red flag symptoms

- Symptoms that require immediate review within 24 h (see Table 13.6)

Table 13.6 **Red flag symptoms for back pain**

RED FLAG SYMPTOMS
• Bladder/bowel changes
• Unexplained weight loss
• Thoracic or non-mechanical
• Age <16 and >50 years
• Bilateral leg pain with neurological symptoms
• Night pain
• History of active or previous malignancy
• Perianal paraesthesia
• Expansile mass
• Chronic steroid use
• Intravenous drug use
• Immunocompromise
• Recent or active infection

Investigations

- Observations: temperature (associated fever)
- Urinalysis: blood, protein ± nitrites, Bence-Jones protein

- Blood tests:
    - FBC: raised WCC in infection and/or inflammation
    - U&E: deranged in renal colic
    - Calcium levels: raised in bony destruction e.g. myeloma
    - Inflammatory markers: raised ESR and CRP
- Blood cultures: if septic patient
- Plain radiograph of spine: unwell and red flags

CAUDA EQUINA SYNDROME

Definition

- Characteristic pattern of neurological and urogenital symptoms due to acute compression of lumbar-sacral nerve roots below the conus medullaris where the spinal cord terminates

Aetiology

- Disc prolapse: most common
- Tumour
- Abscess
- Haematoma
- Trauma

Clinical features

- Back pain
- Radicular pain down both legs
- Leg weakness
- Urinary/faecal incontinence/retention
- ↓ Perianal sensation
- ↓ Anal tone
- LMN signs:
    - ↓ Power
    - ↓ Sensation
    - ↓ Reflexes

Management

- Urgent MRI and neurosurgical review

MICRO-facts

Cauda equina syndrome and rapidly progressing cord compression are emergencies.

Emergency and acute medicine

CORD COMPRESSION

Clinical features

- Lower motor neurone (LMN) signs at level of lesion:
  - ↓ Reflexes
  - ↓ Tone
  - Fasciculations
- Upper motor neurone (UMN) signs below lesion:
  - Spasticity
  - Weakness
  - Hyper-reflexia
  - Upgoing plantars
- Normal findings above level of lesion
- Weakness/numbness of legs
- Pain below lesion
- Incontinence
- Sensation reduced in discrete dermatomal pattern

Investigations

- Urgent MRI spine: lesion

Management

- Immediate referral to orthopaedics/neurosurgeons for urgent decompressive surgery within less than 24 h of symptom onset

Complications

- Permanent neurological damage:
  - Paraplegia
  - Incontinence
  - Weakness
  - Impotence

MECHANICAL BACK PAIN

Aetiology

- Sprain
- Disc prolapse
- Spondylosis

Clinical features

- Pain:
  - Lower back
  - Exacerbated on movement
  - ± Down one leg

- Muscular spasm
- Tender vertebrae
- ± Neurological symptoms

Management
- Analgesia: see Section 1.3
- Early mobilization but avoiding straining, lifting etc.
- Urgent MRI if:
  - No improvement >6 weeks
  - Incontinence
  - Neurological symptoms bilaterally

13.10 ACUTE JOINT PAIN

AETIOLOGY
- Septic arthritis
- Gout/pseudogout
- Osteomyelitis
- Active rheumatoid arthritis
- Seronegative arthritis (rheumatoid factor negative)
- Haemarthrosis
- Reactive arthritis
- Henoch-Schönlein purpura

SEPTIC ARTHRITIS

Definition
- Acute inflammation of a joint due to infection (bacterial or fungal)
- Commonly, single joint: knee or hip affected

Clinical features
- Fever
- Very painful joint
- Monoarthropathy; single joint:
  - Swollen
  - Warm
  - Tender
  - Redness
  - Pain on active and passive movement
  - ↓ Range of movement

Investigations
- Bloods:
  - FBC: ↑ WCC

- Inflammatory markers: raised ESR and CRP
- Blood culture: positive
- Joint aspiration:
  - Microscopy for crystals and cell count
  - Gram stain for organisms
  - Culture
- Plain radiograph of affected joint: destruction of bone, soft tissue damage

> ## MICRO-facts
> Typical organisms cultured from joint aspirate:
> - *Staphylococcus aureus*
> - *Streptococcus pyogenes*
> - *Neisseria gonorrhoeae*

Management

- Analgesia: see Section 1.3
- Urgent orthopaedic referral for joint washout
- High-dose IV antibiotics (triple therapy):
  - 1 g flucloxacillin
  - 1.2 g benzylpenicillin
  - 500 mg metronidazole

ACUTE GOUT

Definition

- Acute inflammatory arthritis with elevated serum uric acid that crystallizes and is deposited into joints

Clinical features

- Severe joint pain
- Swelling
- Erythema and skin appears shiny
- Hot joint
- Gouty tophi
- Most commonly affects first MTPJ
- Past medical history:
  - Minor trauma
  - Previous gout
  - Diet (purines)
  - Alcohol
  - Diuretics – particularly thiazides
  - Low-dose aspirin therapy
  - Renal disease: CKD, stones

Investigations

- Bloods:
  - FBC: raised WCC in inflammation and infection
  - U&E: check renal function
  - Inflammatory markers: raised ESR and CRP
  - Serum uric acid levels (levels may be normal or low in acute attack)
- Blood cultures: if patient has a temperature or septic arthritis suspected
- Joint aspiration:
  - Negatively birefringent crystals
  - Send for culture
- Radiograph of affected joint: soft tissue swelling

MICRO-facts

Pseudogout typically presents similarly to gout with deposition of calcium pyrophosphate crystals, which are weakly positively birefringent on microscopy.

Management

- NSAIDs or colchicine for 2 weeks
- Rest the joint

14 Paediatrics

14.1 ASSESSING THE PAEDIATRIC PATIENT

- See Table 14.1

Principles

- Children are very different to adults.
- Anatomical differences – size and shape.
- Physiological differences – cardiovascular, respiratory and immune function.
- Psychological – emotional response and intellectual ability.
- Weight difference.
- Performing an assessment of an acutely unwell child is different to that of an adult.
- Children cannot always explain their specific complaint and symptoms can often be non-specific.
- Children often have a high physiological reserve, and once they start to decompensate deteriorate very rapidly.
- Always check and double-check drug dosages and calculate according to a child's actual or estimated weight.
- Remember that children and their parents require additional reassurance and explanation.
- Always remember to obtain senior help early.

Paediatric history taking

- Usually taken from parent or guardian in attendance with child
- History of presenting complaint
- Systemic review
    - Cardiovascular:
        - Shortness of breath/sweating especially on feeding
        - Feeding difficulties
        - Cyanosis

Table 14.1 **Assessment of paediatric patients**

ASSESSMENT	CLINICAL FEATURES

Airway and breathing	• ↑ Respiratory rate
	• ↓ Respiratory rate: if exhausted
	• Recessions
	  • Subcostal
	  • Intercostal
	  • Sternal
	• Respiratory noises
	  • Wheezing
	  • Stridor
	  • Grunting
	  • Excretions
	• Accessory muscle use
	  • Head bobbing
	  • Abdominal movement
	  • Shoulder movement
	• Cyanosis
	• Drowsiness
	• Nasal flaring

Circulation	• Tachycardia • Bradycardia (often a pre-terminal sign) • Prolonged capillary refill time (>2 s) • Hypotension • Weak peripheral pulses • ↓ Urine output • Cold peripheries, can often be warm in sepsis • Mottled skin • Agitation/drowsiness
Disability	• ↓ GCS • Drowsiness • Hypotonia • ↓ Blood glucose level

- Respiratory:
  - Shortness of breath
  - Laboured breathing
  - Cough
  - Stridor/wheeze

- Gastrointestinal:
  - Nausea or vomiting
  - Bowel habit: diarrhoea or constipation and description
  - Abdominal pain: often draws knees up to chest
  - Appetite:
    - Avoidance of food
    - Increased thirst – can also occur when the child has a sore throat
  - Weight loss
- Feeding history (baby):
  - Is the baby breast- or bottle-fed?
  - How much, how often?
- Genitourinary (baby): number of wet nappies (helps assess hydration)
- Neurological:
  - Drowsiness
  - Seizures/posturing
  - Headache
- Skin and musculoskeletal:
  - Rash
  - Ulcers
  - Joint pain
- Development: enquire about developmental milestones
- Past medical history
  - Pregnancy and birth history:
    - Complications during pregnancy
    - Gestation at delivery
    - Mode of delivery
    - Any SCBU attendance
  - Previous hospital admissions
- Drug history:
  - Any regular medications
  - Any allergies (both drugs and other allergies including reactions)
- Immunizations: are they up to date?
- Family history:
  - Inherited diseases
  - Health of parents and siblings
- Social history:
  - Who lives at home?
  - Number of siblings
  - Parental circumstances
  - Social care/health visitor involvement
- Review of child health record – the Red Book

Normal values

- See Table 14.2

MICRO-facts

Estimation of a child's weight

$$\text{Weight in kg} = (\text{age} + 4) \times 2$$

Or new APLS calculations:

Age up to 12 months; weight in kg = (1/2 age in months) + 4

Age 1–5 years; weight in kg = (2 × age in years) + 8

Age 5 years and above; weight in kg = (3 × age in years) + 7

Table 14.2 **Normal values in paediatric patients**

AGE	RESPIRATORY RATE/MIN	HEART RATE/MIN	SYSTOLIC BLOOD PRESSURE/MMHG
<1	30–40	110–160	70–90
1–2	25–35	100–150	80–95
2–5	25–30	95–140	80–100
5–12	20–25	80–120	90–110
>12	15–20	60–100	100–120

MICRO-facts

Paracetamol dose:	15 mg/kg 4–6 hourly
Ibuprofen dose:	5 mg/kg 8 hourly

Pain management

- It is important to provide analgesia in unwell children.
- Children rarely tell you they are in pain, but their behaviour often demonstrates this such as becoming quiet and miserable or holding their knees up to their chest.
- Always consult the children's BNF when prescribing for children and calculate dosages according to an actual or estimated weight.

Basic life support

- See Fig. 14.1
- As with any medical emergency, always seek help from senior doctors. Paediatric specialists should be involved as soon as possible.
- Resus Council UK guidelines: available in MICRO-reference.

> **MICRO-reference**
> Paediatric Basic Life Support Guidelines on the Resus Council (UK) website, http://www.resus.org.uk/pages/pbls.pdf

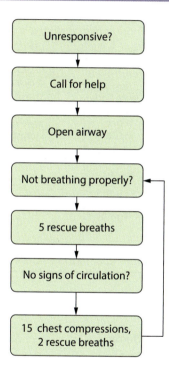

Fig. 14.1 Paediatric Basic Life Support (BLS) algorithm.

Choking management

- See Fig. 14.2

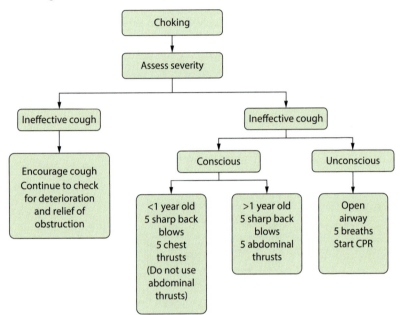

Fig. 14.2 Choking management algorithm.

14.2 RESPIRATORY CONDITIONS

BRONCHIOLITIS

Definition

- Inflammation of the bronchioles

Aetiology

- Respiratory syncytial virus (RSV) (90%)
- Other causes are parainfluenza, influenza, adenoviruses and human metapneumovirus

Clinical features

- Usually occurs in infants <9 months old
- Coryza
- Rhinorrhoea
- Chest cough
- Breathlessness

- Fever
- Poor feeding
- Tachypnoea
- Tachycardia
- Bilateral fine inspiratory crackles with wheeze on auscultation
- Chest hyperinflation with subcostal and intercostal recession

---

MICRO-facts

Risk factors for bronchiolitis

- Age <6 weeks
- Congenital heart disease
- Prematurity
- Respiratory disease
- Immunodeficiency
- Multiple congenital abnormalities
- Severe neurological disease
- Apnoeic episodes

Severity assessment

- See Table 14.3

Table 14.3 **Assessing bronchiolitis severity**

SEVERITY	CLINICAL FEATURES	MANAGEMENT
Mild	• Feeding – well • Respiratory rate <50/min and • SpO_2 >95% on room air • Minimal respiratory distress • No risk factors or social concerns • At least 3 months old	• Monitor at home • Small-volume frequent feeds • Return if deterioration in feeding
Moderate	• Feeding – reduced • Respiratory rate 50–70/min • Mild to moderate respiratory distress • SpO_2 92–95% ORA	• Admit • Oxygen therapy to maintain SpO_2 >95% • Feeding monitoring – may need NG feeds

(Continued)

Table 14.3 *(Continued)* **Assessing bronchiolitis severity**

SEVERITY	CLINICAL FEATURES	MANAGEMENT
Severe	• Poor feeding • Respiratory rate >70 • Moderate to severe respiratory distress • SpO$_2$ 92% on room air • Apnoeic episodes • Unwell/toxic	• Admit to HDU • Consider assisted ventilation • Oxygen therapy to maintain SpO$_2$ >95% • NG feeds

Management

- Supportive
  - Titrated oxygen therapy to maintain SpO$_2$ >95% on room air
  - Monitor:
    - Oxygen saturations
    - Heart rate
- Feeding – NG feeding
- Nasopharyngeal aspirate (NPA) to allow cohort nursing on ward

---

MICRO-case

A 9-month-old female is brought to see her general practitioner by her father. She has had coryzal symptoms for the past 3 days and is becoming increasingly breathless particularly on feeding. Her father reports that she is feeding poorly, miserable and that he can hear her wheezing. On examination she is tachypnoeic, tachycardic with an audible wheeze and end inspiratory crackles on auscultation. She is using her accessory muscles to breathe. The diagnosis of bronchiolitis is made and she is referred to the paediatric team for hospital admission.

Learning points:

- Bronchiolitis is the most common respiratory infection affecting infants <12 months old.
- Annual winter epidemics are common and infants often require hospital admission for supportive treatment.
- Most will recover within 2 weeks.

ASTHMA

Adult asthma is covered in Chapter 4, Respiratory

Clinical features

- See Table 14.4

Table 14.4 **Assessment of asthma severity**

Mild	• SpO$_2$ >95% on room air • Able to talk in full sentences • No respiratory distress
Moderate	• SpO$_2$ 92–95% on room air • Use of accessory muscles • Increased work of breathing
Severe	• Inability to complete sentences or feed • Tachypnoea: >30/min (>5 years) or >40/min (2–5 years) • Tachycardia: >125/min (>5 years) or >140/min (2–5 years) • PEFR 33–50% • Marked respiratory effort • SpO$_2$ <92%

Life threatening	• Remember mnemonic SHOCKED
	  • Silent chest
	  • Hypotension
	  • One-third of best/predicted PEFR (<33%)
	  • Cyanosis
	  • Confusion/coma
	  • K(c)yanosis
	  • Exhaustion – poor respiratory effort
	  • Dysrythmia – bradycardia
	• SpO$_2$ <92%

Management

- Oxygen – high flow 15 L/min via non-rebreathe mask
- Salbutamol:
  - 10 puffs MDI via spacer
  - Via oxygen driven nebulizer
  - 2.5 mg (<5 years) or 5 mg (>5 years)
  - High-dose burst therapy
  - 3 doses back to back
- Ipratropium bromide:
  - 125 mcg (<1 year) or 250 mcg (>1 year) nebulizer
- Steroid:
  - 1-day course oral prednisolone 1–2 mg/kg (40 mg maximum dose)
  - IV hydrocortisone and IV salbutamol if life-threatening
- Hospital admission if:
  - Poor response to treatment
  - ↓ Oxygen saturations <92% on air

Emergency and acute medicine

- Exhaustion
- Severe exacerbations require admission regardless of response to treatment

> **MICRO-reference**
> British Thoracic Society (BTS) and Scottish Intercollegiate Guidelines Network (SIGN) Guidelines on the Management of Asthma, www.sign. ac.uk

CROUP

Definition

- Laryngotracheobronchitis

Aetiology

- Parainfluenza virus

Clinical features

- Children 1–3 years old
- Coryza
- Barking cough
- Harsh stridor
- Mild fever
- Recession

Management

- Clinical severity can be assessed by the Westley modified croup score (Table 14.5)
- Management of croup depends on severity

Table 14.5 **Westley modified croup score**

CLINICAL FEATURE	SEVERITY	SCORE
Chest wall recession	• None	0
	• Mild	1
	• Moderate	2
	• Severe	3
Stridor	• None	0
	• With agitation	1
	• At rest	2

(Continued)

Table 14.5 *(Continued)* **Westley modified croup score**

CLINICAL FEATURE	SEVERITY	SCORE
Cyanosis	• None • With agitation • At rest	0 4 5
Level of consciousness	• Normal • Disorientated	0 5
Air entry	• Normal • Decreased • Markedly decreased	0 1 2

Severity: mild 0–3; moderate 4–6; severe 7–17.

- Mild croup
  - Oral steroids: dexamethasone (0.15 mg/kg to a maximum dose of 10 mg) or prednisolone (2 mg/kg to a maximum dose of 40 mg)
  - Child can be safely discharged from the ED with appropriate instructions.
- Moderate croup
  - May warrant admission depending on clinical progress.
  - Oral steroids as above.
  - If unable to administer steroids orally give 2 mg nebulized budesonide.
- Severe croup
  - Should be assessed and treated in the resuscitation room.
  - Call for senior help immediately.
  - Administer 0.4 mL/g of 1:1000 nebulized adrenaline.
  - Cyanosis at any time indicates severe croup.
  - Intubation may be required.

WHOOPING COUGH

Aetiology

- Respiratory tract infection with *Bordatella pertussis*

Clinical features

- Coryza
- Characteristic cough occurring in paroxysms
- Complications include pneumonia, encephalopathy, seizures and earache

Management

- Refer acutely unwell children to paediatrics
- Erythomycin (12.5 mg/kg QDS) orally: 7-day course
- Avoid contact with other children
- Formal diagnosis confirmed by per nasal swab
- Notifiable disease

INHALED FOREIGN BODY

Key points

- Common in toddlers
- May be anything: food, toys, coins, teeth
- Usually involves right main bronchus as this is more vertical than the left

Clinical features

- Inspiratory stridor
- Wheeze
- Cough

Investigations and management

- Well, relatively asymptomatic:
  - Anterior-posterior chest X-ray
  - Consider lateral neck X-ray if clinical picture consistent with upper airway obstruction
  - Refer to ENT for bronchoscopy
  - Consider anaesthetic assistance
- Complete airway obstruction:
  - Follow Resus Council UK guidelines on choking (Section 14.2)
  - Lower respiratory tract infection

Aetiology and epidemiology

- See Table 14.6

Table 14.6 **Causative organisms of LRTI ordered by age group and prevalence, with most common cause first**

AGE GROUP	CAUSATIVE ORGANISMS
Neonatal	• Group B *Streptococcus* • Listeria monocytogenes • *Staphylococcus aureus* • Gram-negative, e.g. *E. coli*
1 month–2 years	• Viral, e.g. respiratory syncytial virus • *Streptococcus pneumoniae* • *Staphylococcus aureus* • Gram-negative, e.g. *E. coli* • *Chlamydia pneumoniae*
2–5 years	• Viral • *Streptococcus pneumoniae* • *Mycloplasma pneumophila* • *Chlamydia pneumoniae*

(Continued)

Table 14.6 (*Continued*) **Causative organisms of LRTI ordered by age group and prevalence, with most common cause first**

AGE GROUP	CAUSATIVE ORGANISMS
>5 years	• *Mycoplasma pneumoniae* • *Streptococcus pneumoniae* • Viral • *Chlamydia pneumoniae*

> **MICRO-reference**
> British Thoracic Society Standards of Care, British Thoracic Society Guidelines for the Management of Community Acquired Pneumonia in Childhood, *Thorax* 2002:57 (Suppl 1): 1–24.

Clinical features

- Cough
- Fever
- Respiratory distress
- Poor feeding
- Lethargy

Investigations

- CXR: consolidation (Fig. 14.3)

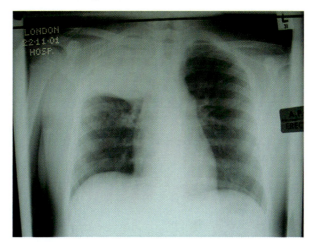

Fig. 14.3 CXR: Right upper lobe consolidation. (From Sidwell, R. and Thompson, M., *Easy Paediatrics*, CRC Press, Boca Raton, FL, 2011.)

Management

- Antibiotics:
  - Type depends on possible organism
  - Route depends on severity
- Supplemental oxygen therapy to maintain SpO_2 above 95%
- Rehydration

14.3 GASTROINTESTINAL AND RENAL TRACT CONDITIONS

ABDOMINAL PAIN

Aetiology

- See Table 14.7

Table 14.7 **Causes of abdominal pain in paediatric patients**

MEDICAL	SURGICAL
• Gastroenteritis	• Acute appendicitis
• Systemic infection	• Intussusception
• Meningitis	• Hirschprung disease
• Local infections	• Incarcerated hernia
• Otitis media	• Ureteric obstruction
• Tonsilitis	• Testicular torsion
• UTI	• Ectopic pregnancy (girls of childbearing age)
• Mesenteric adenitis	• Volvulus
• Coeliac disease	• Malrotation
• Diabetic ketoacidosis	
• Henoch-Schönlein purpura	
• Psychological	
• Non-specific abdominal pain	

Diagnosis and management

- See Chapter 11, Surgical emergencies
- Ascertain an accurate history:
  - Onset
  - Duration
  - Site
- Bowel habit: diarrhoea/constipation

MICRO-facts

Always remember to examine the external genitalia in boys presenting with abdominal pain to rule out testicular torsion.

- Vomiting
- Pyrexia
- Anorexia
- Full examination:
  - Rash
  - Temperature
  - Abdominal distension, tenderness, masses, guarding, bowel sounds
  - Genitalia and hernial orifices
- Obtain urgent surgical review if features of an acute surgical abdomen are present

Investigation

- Bloods:
  - FBC
  - U&E
  - Blood cultures
- Urine dipstick
- Urinary or serum ß-hCG
- Erect CXR: for suspected visceral perforation
- AXR: for suspected bowel obstruction
- USS

Management

- Rehydration
- Analgesia: see Section 1.3
- Antibiotics
- If a surgical abdomen is suspected, keep the patient nil by mouth until surgical review

---

MICRO-case

A 5-year-old boy is brought to the ED by his mother. He has worsening lower abdominal pain over the past 2 h. He had previously been well and playing normally. At present, he is struggling to walk and upset. On examination, his abdomen is soft with lower abdominal tenderness. He has been unable to perform a urine sample for testing. On examination of his genitalia, a tender, erythematous and swollen right testis is found.

Learning points:

- Always examine the external genitalia in boys presenting with abdominal pain.
- Testicular torsion (Fig. 14.1) is an emergency and needs to be relieved within 6 h from symptom onset.
- Refer urgently for a surgical review!
- See also Chapter 11, Surgical emergencies.

Emergency and acute medicine

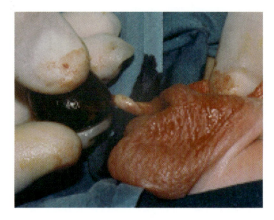

Fig. 14.4 Testicular torsion showing necrotic right testis. (From Sidwell, R. and Thompson, M., *Easy Paediatrics*, CRC Press, Boca Raton, FL, 2011.)

ACUTE APPENDICITIS

Covered in Chapter 11, Surgical emergencies.

MESENTERIC ADENITIS

Definition

- Inflammation of the mesenteric lymph nodes
- Enlarged secondary to a viral or bacterial infection

Clinical features

- Non-localized abdominal pain
- Can often mimic appendicitis

Investigations

- FBC: raised WCC indicates infection
- USS: preferred choice of investigation

Management

- Usually resolves with symptomatic management

INTUSSUSCEPTION

Definition

- Telescoping of one section of intestine into another.
- The blood supply to the distal segment is compromised, which can result in necrosis and perforation.
- Occurs between 6 months and 4 years of age with half of all cases occurring in infants <1 year old with a male:female ratio of 3:1.

Clinical features

- Sudden and episodic abdominal pain
- Drawing up of knees due to pain
- Distressed infant – crying and screaming
- Dehydration
- Abdominal distension
- Abdominal tenderness and palpable 'sausage' mass
- Vomiting
- 'Redcurrant jelly' stool – late sign

Investigations

- AXR: may show signs of bowel obstruction
- Air or barium enema:
  - Is also curative
  - Not to be performed if peritonitic

Management

- Resuscitation – IV fluids
- Urgent surgical referral for reduction

INTESTINAL OBSTRUCTION

Aetiology

- Pyloric stenosis
- Intussusception
- Appendicitis
- Inguinal hernia
- Inflammatory bowel disease
- Volvulus
- Malrotation

Clinical features

- Abdominal distension
- Abdominal tenderness
- Absolute constipation
- Hyperactive bowel sounds
- Vomiting
- Features of shock

Management

- Resuscitation – IV fluids
- Nil by mouth, NGT
- Analgesia
- Urgent surgical review – treat cause of obstruction

Emergency and acute medicine

14.4 DIARRHOEA AND VOMITING

Aetiology

- See Table 14.8

Table 14.8 **Causes of diarrhoea and vomiting in paediatric patients**

MEDICAL	SURGICAL

• Gastroenteritis
• Systemic infection:
  • Meningitis
• Local infections:
  • Otitis media
  • Tonsillitis
  • UTI
• Coeliac disease
• Diabetic ketoacidosis
• Psychological
	• Acute appendicitis
	• Intussusception
	• Hirschprung disease

MICRO-facts

Diarrhoea and vomiting are very common and not always due to gastroenteritis. Always perform a full examination to rule out other causes.

MICRO-facts

Viral gastroenteritis is unlikely if the following are present:

- Bloody diarrhoea
- Severe abdominal pain
- Bilious vomiting
- Septicaemia

Consider more serious causes such as acute abdominal pathology.

Investigations

- FBC: raised WCC
- U&E: renal function
- Imaging: if clinically indicated
- Stool culture: if clinically indicated

Management
- Rehydration: oral or IV fluids depending on severity
- Antibiotics if indicated

14.5 DEHYDRATION

Clinical features and severity assessment
- See Table 14.9

Table 14.9 **Assessing severity of dehydration**

DEHYDRATION SEVERITY	CLINICAL FEATURES
Mild <5%	• Well • Increased thirst • Slight reduction in urine output
Moderate 5–10%	• Unwell • Restless • Sunken eyes and fontanelle • Tachycardia • Tachypnoea • Normal capillary refill time • Oliguria • Reduced skin turgor • Dry mucous membranes • Normal blood pressure
Severe >10%	• Drowsy • Cold, pale mottled skin • Weak peripheral pulses • Hypotension • Marked oliguria • Prolonged capillary refill time • Tachycardia • Tachypnoea • Decreased level of consciousness

Management
- Fluid rehydration (see Fig. 14.5):
  - Replace fluid deficit (see MICRO-facts box for calculation)
  - Replace ongoing losses
  - Provide maintenance fluid (see Table 14.10)

Emergency and acute medicine

> ## MICRO-facts
> Calculating fluid deficit in mL = % dehydration × body weight (kg) × 10

Table 14.10 **Calculating fluid maintenance**

BODY WEIGHT	FLUID MAINTENANCE ML/KG/24 H
First 10 kg	100
Second 10 kg	50
Each subsequent kg	20

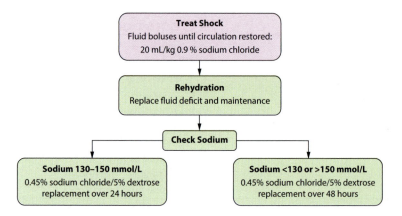

Fig. 14.5 Calculating fluid rehydration.

14.6 THE FEBRILE CHILD

Definition
- Temperature >38.0°C

Aetiology
- See Table 14.11

Clinical features
- Lethargy
- Poor feeding
- Miserable
- Signs of dehydration
- Reduced urinary output
- Tachycardia

Table 14.11 **Causes of a febrile child**

SYSTEM	AETIOLOGY
Respiratory	• Upper respiratory tract infection • Lower respiratory tract infection • Croup
Gastrointestinal	• Gastroenteritis • Appendicitis
ENT	• Otitis media • Tonsillitis • Epiglottitis
Genitourinary	• Lower urinary tract infection • Upper urinary tract infection
Neurological	• Meningitis • Encephalitis • Seizure
Other	• Osteomyelitis • Septic arthritis • Kawasaki disease • Septicaemia, e.g. meningococcal

- Hypotension
- Tachypnoea/respiratory distress
- Fever
- Purpuric rash – meningococcal septicaemia
- Hypoxia/cyanosis
- Joint/limb swelling

Investigations: Septic screen

- Bloods:
  - FBC: May show raised WCC indicating infection
  - Glucose
  - U&Es: raised urea and creatinine can indicate dehydration
  - Blood cultures
  - Acute phase reactants: ↑ CRP and ESR
- Meningococcal PCR
- Throat swab
- Urine for microscopy, culture and sensitivity
- CXR: rule out pneumonia
- Lumbar puncture: if indicated would be performed by the paediatric team

Management

- Treat the cause if a focus of infection is found
- Admit if:
    - Systemically unwell, with or without focus of infection
    - 0–3 months old with a temperature >38°C
    - 3–6 months old with a temperature >39°C
    - Signs of meningism (see below)
    - Non-blanching rash
- Discharge if:
    - No systemic toxic findings
    - No abnormalities in septic screen
    - Infection may be safely managed at home:
        - Regular fluid intake
        - Paracetamol
        - Ibuprofen
        - Antibiotics if indicated
        - Review with GP in 24–48 h, or sooner if any concerns

14.7 FEBRILE CONVULSIONS

Definition

- Seizure occurring in a child from 6 months to 5 years who is neurologically normal precipitated by a fever arising from infection outside the nervous system

Epidemiology

- 6 months–5 years
- Affects 3% of children
- Can often reoccur

Clinical features

- Typically last <5 min but may develop into a complex febrile seizure lasting >15 min
- No focal neurological deficit
- No residual weakness

Investigations

- Septic screen: see Section 14.6

Management

- Treat underlying aetiology
- Manage convulsion (see Table 14.12)
- Reduce the fever (see Table 14.12)

Table 14.12 **Management of febrile convulsions**

Manage the convulsion	• Oxygen • IV lorazepam (0.1 mg/kg) or PR diazepam (0.5 mg/kg) if appropriate
Reduce the fever	• Undress • Tepid sponging/fan • Paracetamol • Ibuprofen • Treat cause

- Admit if:
  - First febrile seizure
  - <2 years old
- Discuss with paediatric team if any concerns

14.8 MENINGITIS AND MENINGOCOCCAL SEPTICAEMIA

> **MICRO-facts**
>
> Bacterial meningitis carries a 5–10% mortality rate.

Aetiology

- May be due to bacteria or viruses
- Enterovirus accounts for 80% of viral meningitis
- See Table 14.13 for bacterial epidemiology
- If in doubt as to the cause, always treat as bacterial, as more likely to cause complications

Key points

- Meningitis:
  - Inflammation of the meningeal tissues that surround the brain
  - Refer to Chapter 18, Infectious diseases
- Meningococcal septicaemia:
  - Septicaemia caused by *Neisseria meningitidis*
  - May or may not be associated with meningitis
  - Carries a high risk of complication and mortality

Emergency and acute medicine

Table 14.13 **Causative organisms in meningitis**

AGE	CAUSATIVE ORGANISM
Neonatal–3 months	• Group B *Streptococcus* • *Listeria monocytogenes* • *Escherichia coli*
1 month–6 years	• *Neisseria meningitidis* • *Streptococcus pneumoniae* • *Haemophilus influenzae*
Over 6 years	• *Neisseria. meningitidis* • *S. pneumoniae*

History

- Fever, rigors
- Irritability, confusion
- Lethargy, drowsiness
- Headache
- Photophobia
- Vomiting
- Seizures

Examination

- Early signs are often non-specific
- Fever
- Features of meningism:
  - Neck stiffness
  - Brudzinski sign
  - Kernig sign

MICRO-facts

- Brudzinski sign: With the child supine, neck flexion causes flexion of the knees and hips.
- Kernig sign: With the child supine, hips and knees flexed, extension of the knees causes back pain.

- Features of shock:
  - Tachycardia
  - Prolonged capillary refill time
  - Tachypnoea
  - Drowsiness
  - Reduced urine output
  - Hypotension (late sign)

- Features of raised intracranial pressure:
    - Fluctuating or reduced consciousness
    - Relative bradycardia and hypertension
    - Unequal, dilated pupils
    - Seizures
    - Focal neurological signs
- Features of septicaemia:
    - Shock (see above)
    - Purpuric, non-blanching rash (late sign, may be atypical)

Investigations

- Blood tests:
    - FBC
    - U&Es
    - LFT
    - Clotting screen
    - CRP
    - Blood cultures (take before starting antibiotics)
    - Meningococcal PCR
- Other microbiology:
    - Urine
    - Throat swab
    - Stool
- Lumbar puncture
- CT/MRI if appropriate; do not allow to delay treatment

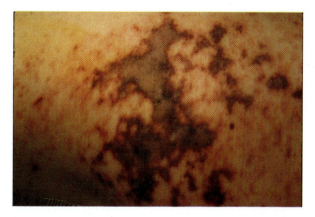

Fig. 14.6 Petechial rash. (From Sidwell, R. and Thompson, M., *Easy Paediatrics*, CRC Press, Boca Raton, FL, 2011.)

Emergency and acute medicine

Management

- See Fig. 14.7

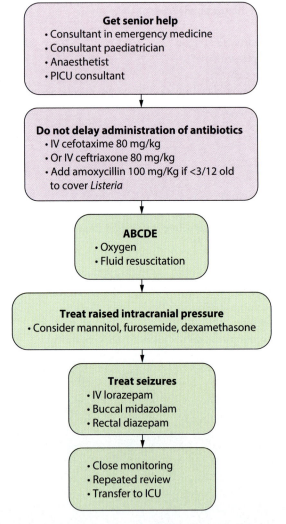

Fig. 14.7 Emergency management of meningococcal septicaemia.

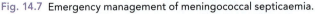

MICRO-reference
NICE Guidelines on Management of Bacterial Meningitis and
Meningococcal Septicaemia, http://guidance.nice.org.uk/CG102

14.9 SKIN CONDITIONS

RASHES

- See Table 14.14

ATOPIC ECZEMA

Clinical features

- Dry, itchy skin
- Skin flexures (see Fig. 14.8)
- Frictional areas
- Family or personal history of atopy (asthma, eczema, allergic rhinitis) is common

Management

- Emollient cream
- Anti-pruritic: antihistamines
- Steroid cream:
  - 0.5–1% hydrocortisone twice daily
  - Avoid potent preparations on the face
- Consider systemic or topical antibiotics if evidence of superimposed infection
- Advise to avoid irritants
- Arrange dermatology follow-up if severe

Table 14.14 **Skin rashes and causes**

CHARACTERISTIC	AETIOLOGY
Itchy	• Atopic eczema • Urticaria • Scabies • Chicken pox • Fungal infections
Petechial	• Meningococcal disease • Henoch-Schönlein purpura • Idiopathic thrombocytopenia • Viral illness • Trauma • Superior vena cava distribution
Blistering	• Chicken pox • Herpes zoster • Hand, foot and mouth disease • Stevens-Johnson syndrome

Emergency and acute medicine

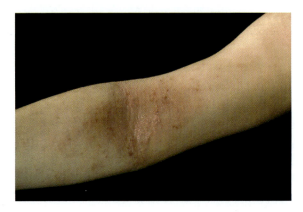

Fig. 14.8 Flexural eczema. (From Sidwell, R. and Thompson, M., *Easy Paediatrics*, CRC Press, Boca Raton, FL, 2011.)

URTICARIA

Aetiology
- Hypersensitivity
- May be due to specific allergens

Clinical features
- Hives, wheals, flares (see Fig. 14.9)
- Oedematous lesions
- Angioedema

Management
- Antihistamines, e.g. chlorphenamine
- Emollient cream
- Management of anaphylaxis, if present (see Section 1.2)
- Adrenaline doses in children:
    - >12 years: 500 micrograms IM (0.5 mL) i.e. same as adult dose
    - >6 – 12 years: 300 micrograms IM (0.3 mL)
    - >6 months – 6 years: 150 micrograms IM (0.15 mL)
    - <6 months: 150 micrograms IM (0.15 mL)
- Avoid allergens
- Dermatology follow-up

HENOCH-SCHÖNLEIN PURPURA (HSP)

Definition
- Systemic vasculitis affecting the small arterioles of the skin, joints, gastrointestinal tract and kidneys

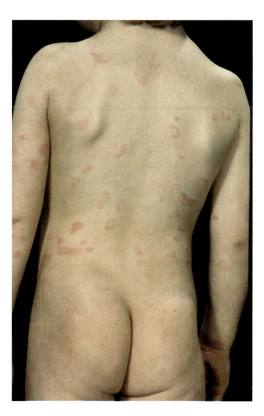

Fig. 14.9 Urticaria wheals. (From Sidwell, R. and Thompson, M., *Easy Paediatrics*, CRC Press, Boca Raton, FL, 2011.)

Aetiology

- Follows a recent viral or bacterial illness, e.g. upper respiratory tract infection or gastroenteritis
- More common in boys
- Usually affects children aged 2–11 years

Clinical features

- Rash:
    - Characteristically over buttocks/extensor surfaces of limbs (Fig. 14.10)
    - Symmetrical
    - Maculopapular
    - Purpuric or petechial
- Nephritis:
    - Oedema
    - Abdominal pain

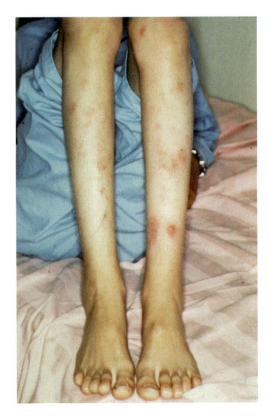

Fig. 14.10 Henoch-Schönlein purpura. (From Sidwell, R. and Thompson, M., *Easy Paediatrics*, CRC Press, Boca Raton, FL, 2011.)

- Haematuria
- Proteinuria
- Hypertension
- Arthralgia:
  - ± Joint swelling typically affecting the larger joints lasting up to 48 h

Investigation

- Visual inspection of urine for macroscopic haematuria
- Urine dipstick for blood ± microscopy to quantify RBC count
- Measure blood pressure
- Further investigations as dictated by degree of systemic upset, haematuria or hypertension

Management

- Supportive management of above symptoms: analgesia
- Assess for renal damage: renal history

SCABIES

Aetiology

- Infestation with *Sarcoptes scabiei*

Clinical features

- Severe itching
- Burrows between fingers but can occur in other flexure surfaces
- See Fig. 14.11

Management

- Treat both the patient and their household contacts
- 5% permethrin cream applied everywhere below the neck for 8–12 h

HAND-FOOT-AND-MOUTH DISEASE

Aetiology

- Molluscum contagiosum virus

Clinical features

- Pearly papules
- Affecting hands, feet and mucous membranes of the mouth
- Parents may report that other children in contact have the virus
- See Fig. 14.12

Management

- Self-limiting, no specific treatment required
- Advise parents to keep child away from other children until the rash has cleared

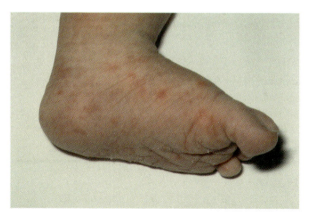

Fig. 14.11 Scabies. (From Sidwell, R. and Thompson, M., *Easy Paediatrics*, CRC Press, Boca Raton, FL, 2011.)

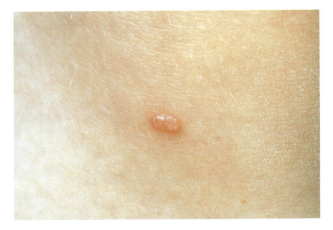

Fig. 14.12 Molluscum contagiosum. (From Sidwell, R. and Thompson, M., *Easy Paediatrics*, CRC Press, Boca Raton, FL, 2011.)

VARICELLA ZOSTER (CHICKEN POX)

Aetiology

- Varicella zoster virus
- Incubation period of 10–21 days

Management

- Supportive and symptomatic, e.g. paracetamol, calamine lotion, oral antihistamines
- Avoid NSAIDs: increased risk of developing invasive streptococcal disease
- Consider the following in severe cases:
  - Admission
  - Varicella zoster immunoglobulin
  - Aciclovir

Complications

- Secondary bacterial infection
- Pneumonia/pneumonitis
- Cerebellar ataxia
- Hepatitis
- Encephalitis

> ## MICRO-facts
>
> There has been a sharp increase in the number of cases of measles in recent years. This is most likely due to the false claim that linked the MMR vaccine to autism.

MEASLES

Aetiology

- Highly infectious RNA paramyxovirus
- Droplet transmission
- Most common in children aged 1–4 years old

Clinical features

- Prodromal stage:
  - Cough
  - Coryza
  - Conjunctivitis
  - Koplik spots: white spots on mucous membranes of mouth
  - Infective during this stage until fourth day of rash
- Rash:
  - Maculopapular red rash (see Fig. 14.13)
  - Spreads downwards from face

Complications

- Otitis media
- Diarrhoea
- Secondary bacterial infection, e.g. pneumonia, cellulitis
- Meningitis
- Encephalitis
- Subacute sclerosing panencephalitis
- Complications during pregnancy if infected while pregnant

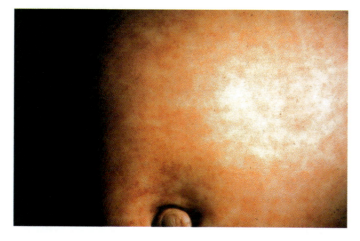

Fig. 14.13 Measles rash. (From Sidwell, R. and Thompson, M., *Easy Paediatrics*, CRC Press, Boca Raton, FL, 2011.)

Emergency and acute medicine

Management

- Symptomatic:
  - Analgesia
  - Monitor fluid balance
  - Treat any secondary infection
- Immunoglobulin can be used in infants and immunocompromised patients within 6 days of exposure

MUMPS

Aetiology

- RNA paramyxovirus
- Droplet transmission

Clinical features

- Prodomal stage:
  - Non-specific symptoms
  - Fever
  - Myalgia
  - Headache
- Tender swelling of salivary glands, mainly parotid

Complications

- Meningitis
- Encephalitis
- Epididymo-orchitis
- Eye symptoms
- Pancreatitis

Management

- Symptomatic: analgesia
- Management of above complications

RUBELLA

Aetiology

- RNA togavirus
- Droplet transmission

Clinical features

- Prodomal stage:
  - Non-specific symptoms
  - Fever
  - Coryza
  - Myalgia
  - Headache

- Pink maculopapular rash:
  - Spreads downwards from face
- Cervical lymphadenopathy

Complications

- Teratogenic in pregnancy:
  - Fetal complications worst during first trimester
  - Congenital rubella syndrome
- Arthritis
- Encephalitis
- Thrombocytopaenia

Management

- Supportive
- Obstetric advice if pregnant

14.10 EAR, NOSE AND THROAT

TONSILLITIS AND PHARYNGITIS

Covered in Chapter 16, Ear, nose and throat

MICRO-facts

NICE Centor criteria for sore throat
- Tonsillar exudate
- Absence of cough
- History of fever
- Tender anterior cervical lymph nodes

Presence of three or four clinical signs suggests chance of patient having group A β-haemolytic streptococcal infection is 40–60% and so may benefit from antibiotic treatment.

OTITIS MEDIA

Covered in Chapter 16, Ear, nose and throat

EPIGLOTTITIS

Definition

- Inflammation of the epiglottis

Aetiology

- Haemophilus influenzae type B

Epidemiology

- Usually 1 to 6 years old

Clinical features

- Acute onset
- Toxic, septic, unwell
- Difficulty talking
- Drooling saliva
- Respiratory distress
- Open mouth
- Upright in a 'tripod' position to aid accessory muscle use
- Stridor

MICRO-facts

Remember epiglottitis
- Sepsis
- Stridor
- Saliva – drooling
- Speech – muffled
- Swallowing – difficult

Management

- Urgent senior ENT, anaesthetic and paediatric help required to secure airway.
- Do not attempt bloods or cannulation until the airway is secure, as this can cause the child to become distressed and further compromise the airway.
- Intravenous antibiotics – cefotaxime if not allergic.

MICRO-facts

Never examine the throat in suspected epiglottitis as this may further compromise the airway!

Acute epiglottitis vs. croup

- See Table 14.15

Table 14.15 **Acute epiglottitis vs. croup**

FEATURE	CROUP	EPIGLOTTITIS
Onset	Days	Hours
Preceeding coryza	Yes	No

(Continued)

Table 14.15 *(Continued)* **Acute epiglottitis vs. croup**

FEATURE	CROUP	EPIGLOTTITIS
Cough	Severe Barking	Absent Slight
Able to drink	Yes	No
Drooling saliva	No	Yes
Appearance	Unwell	Toxic/very unwell
Fever	<38.5	>38.5
Stridor	Harsh Rasping	Soft Whispering
Voice/cry	Hoarse	Muffled Reluctant to speak
Pain	Not usually	Intensely painful

14.11 URINARY TRACT INFECTION (UTI)

See also Chapter 8, Renal emergencies.

Definition

- Pure growth of 10^4–10^5 organisms/mL

Clinical features

- Non-specific symptoms:
  - Poor feeding
  - Lethargy
  - Irritable
- Pyrexia
- Dysuria
- Offensive-smelling urine
- Abdominal pain
- Incontinence

MICRO-facts

- Symptoms of a UTI can be non-specific especially in children under 3 years.
- Always remember to test urine samples in children with an unexplained fever.

Diagnosis

- Clean catch urine dipstick, presence of:
  - Nitrites (highly indicative)
  - Leucocytes
  - Blood
  - Protein
- Positive urine culture, confirms UTI

> **MICRO-facts**
>
> Measure BP, height, weight and temperature in all children presenting with a UTI. Abnormalities in these readings may suggest underlying pathology.

Management

- Infants <3 months must be admitted
- Children >3 months with symptoms of a lower urinary tract infection can be treated with 3 days of oral antibiotics
- Treat with antibiotics if clinical features and urine dipstick are suggestive of a UTI
- Antibiotic choice can be based on local guidelines; trimethoprim, amoxicillin, cephalosporin and nitrofurantoin may all be suitable
- Hydration
- Re-assess the child after 24–48 h if still unwell
- Further investigations may be needed to check for any renal structural abnormalities

> **MICRO-references**
>
> NICE Guidelines (CG54) on Urinary Tract Infection; Diagnosis, Treatment and Long Term Management of Urinary Tract Infection in Children, www.nice.org.uk/CG54

14.12 THE LIMPING CHILD

Aetiology

- Wide differential diagnoses:
  - Medical causes:
    - Neoplasia
    - Sickle cell disease
    - Leukaemia
    - Sepsis
  - Non-accidental injury (NAI)

- Bony/joint causes:
  - Septic arthritis
  - Fracture
  - Osteomyelitis
  - Soft tissue injury
  - Discitis
- Hip pathologies:
  - Transient synovitis
  - Most common presentation especially following active or recent URTI
  - Perthes disease
  - Septic arthritis
  - Slipped upper femoral epiphysis
  - Missed developmental dysplasia of the hip
- Surgical:
  - Peritonitis
  - Hernias
  - Testicular torsion

14.13 THE HYPOGLYCAEMIC (NON-DIABETIC) CHILD

Definition
- Hypoglycaemia:
  - May be the only presenting complaint for a serious underlying metabolic condition
  - Plasma glucose less than 2.5 mmol/L
  - Threshold definitions vary from hospital to hospital; follow local hospital policy

Management
- Hypoglycaemic screening blood tests prior to giving glucose
- Neonates <72 h who are yet to establish feeding:
  - Observe response after single feed
  - Consider hypoglycaemic screening blood tests
  - Refer to the paediatric team for admission

14.14 NON-ACCIDENTAL INJURY AND ABUSE

Definition
- Parents or carers can inflict abuse on children under their care in different forms:
  - Physical

Emergency and acute medicine

- Emotional
- Sexual
- Neglect

Recognition

- History:
    - May not be consistent with injuries sustained
    - Denial of injury
    - Changing, variable
    - Unexplained delay in presentation
    - Frequent ED attendance
    - Missed appointments for medical care
- Examination:
    - Parental interaction
    - Injuries inconsistent with the child's developmental stage
    - Old injuries
    - Failure to thrive
    - Quiet, watchful child
    - Delay in developmental milestones
    - Unusual sites for injuries:
        - Face
        - Back
        - Thigh
    - Specific injuries:
        - Bite marks
        - Finger marks
        - Burns
        - Torn frenulum
        - Retinal haemorrhages
        - Trauma to genitalia
        - Fractures in a child <2 years old
    - Sexually transmitted infections
    - Fabricated or induced illness

MICRO-facts

Don't forget medical causes. Immune thrombocytopenic purpura (ITP) can also present with multiple bruises and petechiae and osteogenesis imperfecta with fractures.

Management

- Inform senior member of ED.
- Inform senior paediatrician.
- Arrange admission to enable further investigation, observation and safeguarding procedures to be instituted.
- Check the child protection register to see if previous episodes of abuse have been recorded.
- Document clearly and accurately.

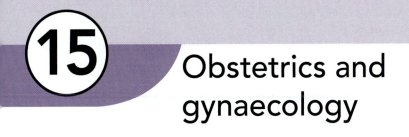

15 Obstetrics and gynaecology

15.1 THE PREGNANT PATIENT

Definitions

- Gravidity: total number of pregnancies
- Parity: number of times given birth to a foetus with gestational age >24 weeks

Management

- Can cause considerable anxiety to patient and doctor
- Always elicit senior/obstetric help when in doubt
- Try to avoid X-rays and CT scans due to potential radiation risk to foetus unless absolutely necessary (discuss with a senior)
- Always consult BNF prior to prescribing

15.2 EMERGENCY DELIVERY

Clinical features

- After 24th week gestation
- Painful uterine contractions
- Cervical dilatation >3 cm
- Rupture of membranes

Assessment

- ABCDE
- Palpate abdomen
- Auscultate foetal heart using Pinard stethoscope or handheld Doppler

Management

- Call obstetric and neonatal teams immediately
- Analgesia
- Ask mother to take short, shallow breaths
- Control delivery of head once crowned
- Palpate for umbilical cord wrapped around neck, and gently slip off if felt

- Allow delivery of the anterior shoulder followed by the posterior shoulder and trunk
- Syntometrine IM (oxytocin 5 units with ergometrine 500 µg) or oxytocin 10 units administered with birth of the anterior shoulder
- Clamp and cut umbilical cord once pulsation ceases if condition of baby allows
- Dry and wrap baby and pass to mother (if condition and gestational age allows) before handing to the paediatrician
- Wait for signs of placental separation and deliver placenta
- Check uterus is well contracted and blood loss normal
- Inspect perineum for any tears or lacerations and treat appropriately

15.3 VAGINAL BLEEDING IN PREGNANCY

Aetiology

- See Table 15.1

Table 15.1 **Causes of vaginal bleeding in pregnancy**

TIME IN PREGNANCY	CAUSE OF BLEEDING
Early <24 weeks	• Ectopic pregnancy • Miscarriage
Late >24 weeks	• Placental abruption • Placenta praevia • Vasa praevia • Uterine rupture
Anytime	• Infection • Trauma • Coagulation disorders • Vaginal pathology • Cervical pathology

Clinical features according to aetiology

- See Table 15.2

Table 15.2 **Clinical features and causes of vaginal bleeding**

CAUSE	CLINICAL FEATURES
Ectopic pregnancy	• Abdominal pain • Vaginal bleeding • Often amenorrhoea • Collapse/syncope

(Continued)

Table 15.2 *(Continued)* **Clinical features and causes of vaginal bleeding**

CAUSE	CLINICAL FEATURES

Miscarriage	• Threatened:
	  • Abdominal cramps
	  • Vaginal bleeding
	  • Closed cervical os
	• Inevitable
	  • Persistent abdominal cramps
	  • Heavier vaginal bleeding
	  • Open cervical os
	• Complete
	  • All foetal products expelled
	  • Closed cervical os
	• Incomplete
	  • Abdominal cramps
	  • Heavy vaginal bleeding
	  • Retained products of conception
	  • Products can become infected → septic miscarriage
	• Missed
	  • Early in pregnancy
	  • Retained products
	  • Brownish vaginal discharge

Placental abruption	• Abdominal pain • Vaginal bleeding, but can often be concealed bleeding • Hard, tender, woody uterus
Placenta praevia	• Often painless vaginal bleeding • Sometimes mild abdominal cramps

15.4 ECTOPIC PREGNANCY

Definition

- Implantation of embryo outside the uterus
- Most common location is the fallopian tubes

Risk factors

- Pelvic inflammatory disease (PID)
- Intrauterine contraceptive device (IUCD)
- Previous fallopian tubal surgery
- IVF treatment
- Previous ectopic pregnancy

> **MICRO-facts**
>
> Consider ectopic pregnancy in females with:
> - Abdominal pain
> - Collapse/syncope
> - Menstrual irregularities
> - Vaginal bleeding
>
> Always do a pregnancy test!

Investigations

- Serum and urinary β-hCG
- Request rhesus status: may need anti-D immunoglobulin if mother rhesus negative
- Cross-match 6 units of blood
- Transabdominal or transvaginal pelvic ultrasound scan

Management

- Inform gynaecologist and anaesthetist
- Resuscitation, if required

15.5 MISCARRIAGE

Clinical features

- See Table 15.2

Management

- Inform gynaecologist
- Resuscitation: if required
- 500 μg of ergometrine IM: if severe bleeding
- Check rhesus status

15.6 PLACENTAL ABRUPTION

Definition

- Premature separation of the placenta from the uterine wall

Risk factors

- Smoking
- Previous placental abruption
- Pre-eclampsia
- Trauma

Investigations

- Cross-match
- Check rhesus status
- Abdominal ultrasound scan

> **MICRO-facts**
>
> In rhesus-negative patients give anti-D immunoglobulin 250 units IM. This will prevent maternal formation of antibodies.

Management

- Inform obstetrician
- Never perform a vaginal examination:
  - Can precipitate further bleeding
  - Should only be performed by an experienced obstetrician
- Left lateral position
- Resuscitation

15.7 PLACENTA PRAEVIA

Definition

- Low-lying placenta

Risk factors

- High parity
- Previous placenta praevia
- Uterine abnormalities e.g. fibroids

Management

- Inform obstetrician
- Never perform a vaginal examination
- Resuscitation

15.8 VASA PRAEVIA

Definition

- Abnormal foetal blood vessels present near the internal os

Clinical features

- Bleeding more common during labour

> **MICRO-case**
>
> A 25-year-old woman who is 30 weeks pregnant presents with a 2-day history of worsening achy lower abdominal pain. She has been having urinary frequency, dysuria and offensive-smelling urine. A urinary dip is positive for nitrites and leucocytes. A 3-day course of amoxicillin is given for a lower urinary tract infection.
>
> **Learning points:**
>
> - UTIs are more common in pregnancy due to urinary stasis and dilation of the upper renal tract.
> - UTIs are an important cause of premature labour and should be treated.
> - Always remember to consult the BNF when prescribing for pregnant women!

15.9 HYPEREMESIS GRAVIDARUM

Definition

- Excessive vomiting in pregnancy resulting in severe dehydration
- Usually subsides by the second trimester

Risk factors

- Multiple pregnancy
- Molar pregnancy
- Urinary tract infection
- Hyperthyroidism

Clinical features

- Vomiting
- Fatigue
- Reduced appetite
- Electrolyte disturbance
- Weight loss

Investigations

- Bloods:
  - FBC
  - U&E
  - TFTs
- Urine dipstick: presence of urinary ketones indicates severity of dehydration

Management

- IV fluids
- IV antiemetics

- Vitamin B$_1$ (thiamine) supplementation:
  - Can be lost in severe vomiting
  - Prevents Wernicke encephalopathy

15.10 PRE-ECLAMPSIA AND ECLAMPSIA

Definition
- Hypertension: ≥140/90
- Proteinuria: ≥300 mg in 24 h

Risk factors
- Previous pre-eclampsia
- Extremes of age
- Multiple pregnancies
- Diabetes
- Hypertension

Clinical features
- Hypertension
- Proteinuria
- Headache
- Abdominal pain
- Oedema
- Nausea
- Confusion

> **MICRO-facts**
>
> Pre-eclampsia can present as RUQ abdominal pain. Remember to check:
> - BP
> - Urine dipstick for proteinuria

Complications
- Eclampsia: seizures
- HELLP:
  - Haemolysis
  - Elevated liver enzymes
  - Low platelets
- DIC
- Placental abruption
- Renal failure

Emergency and acute medicine

Management

- Inform obstetrician immediately
- ABCDE approach to resuscitation
- Bloods:
  - FBC: low platelets and anaemia may be present
  - U&E: renal failure can occur
  - Glucose
  - LFTs: can be deranged
  - Clotting screen: can be deranged
  - Uric acid: may be raised
- Left lateral position
- Strict fluid balance chart
- For seizure prophylaxis and eclampsia – IV magnesium sulphate: check local hospital policy
- Treat severe hypertension: IV labetalol 10 mg slow infusion
- Urgent deliver

15.11 MENORRHAGIA

Definition

- Heavy uterine bleeding

Aetiology

- Fibroids
- Dysfunctional uterine bleeding (DUB)
- Endometriosis
- Pelvic inflammatory disease (PID)
- Thyroid dysfunction

Management

- Resuscitate if necessary
- Cross-match and check FBC, clotting screen
- Dependent on severity:
  - Inpatient management:
    - Inform gynaecologist
  - Outpatient management:
    - Less severe
    - Not haemodynamically compromised
    - Hb within normal limits
    - Mefenamic acid 500 mg TDS for pain of DUB
    - Tranexamic acid 1 g TDS for DUB
    - GP follow-up

MICRO-case

A 45-year-old woman presents to the ED feeling tired, light-headed and complaining of heavy menstrual bleeding. She is on the second day of her period and has needed to change her sanitary towel every 2 h. She is passing clots, and is very concerned as this period is particularly heavier than usual. She has no medical history of note and takes no contraception.

She is hypotensive at 90/60 mmHg and tachycardic at 110 bpm. Pregnancy is ruled out, and blood tests reveal a Hb of 6 g/dL. She is resuscitated and given 1 g of tranexamic acid. She is cross-matched and transfused 4 units of blood and admitted under the care of the gynaecology team. During her inpatient stay a transvaginal ultrasound scan reveals submucosal fibroids.

Learning points:
- Always rule out pregnancy in females of a reproductive age.
- In females above 40 years, endometrial pathology should always be excluded.
- Always check FBC, clotting screen, TFTs; results can often be surprising!
- Menorrhagia is common at extremes of age.

15.12 GYNAECOLOGICAL PAIN

PELVIC INFLAMMATORY DISEASE

Definition
- Endometritis
- Salpingitis
- Oophoritis
- Peritonitis
- Acute or chronic

Aetiology
- *Chlamydia trachomatis*
- *Neisseria gonorrhoea*
- *Mycoplasma genitalium*

Clinical features
- Fever
- Malaise
- Bilateral lower abdominal tenderness
- Abnormal vaginal discharge
- Cervical and adnexal tenderness on PV examination

Emergency and acute medicine

Investigations

- Serum/urinary β-hCG
- Urinalysis
- Triple swabs
- Blood cultures, infective markers

Management

- Discharge with antibiotics; if stable:
  - Ofloxacin 400 mg twice daily and metronidazole 400 mg twice daily for 14 days with GUM clinic follow-up and contact tracing
- Admission required if:
  - Uncertain diagnosis
  - Vomiting
  - Suspected tubo-ovarian mass
  - Temperature greater than 38°C
  - Septic/systemically unwell
  - Uncontrolled abdominal/pelvic pain

ENDOMETRIOSIS

Definition

- Presence of endometrial tissue in the pelvis outside the uterus

Clinical features

- Abdominal pain, flank pain worse pre-menstrually and menstrually
- Dysmenorrhoea
- Dyspareunia
- Infertility

MICRO-facts

Endometriosis
- 2–50% cases have no symptoms
- Pain is often non-specific and can result in a delayed diagnosis

---

Management

- Analgesia
- Gynaecology outpatient follow-up or admission if severe uncontrolled symptoms

15.13 EMERGENCY CONTRACEPTION

Medications used

- Levonorgestrel – Levonelle® 1500 (1.5 mg) as soon as possible but within 72 h of unprotected sexual intercourse
- Ulipristal acetate – ellaOne® as soon as possible but within 120 h of unprotected sexual intercourse
- IUCD insertion up to 5 days after unprotected intercourse
- May also need HIV post-exposure prophylaxis/hepatitis B accelerated immunization regimen/stored sample

Contraindications

- Acute porphyria
- Pregnancy
- Severe liver disease
- Previous allergy/intolerance

Advice

- If vomits within 3 h will need replacement dose
- Follow up with GP/GUM clinic
- Future contraception
- If next period delayed or abnormal need to perform pregnancy test

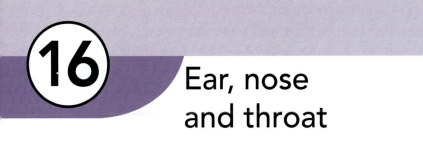

Ear, nose and throat

16.1 THE EAR

OTITIS EXTERNA

Definition

- Inflammation and infection of the epithelial lining of the external auditory canal

Aetiology

- *Staphylococcus aureus*
- *Pseudomonas aeruginosa*

Risk factors

- Underlying skin disease – eczema
- Diabetes
- Swimming

Clinical features

- Tender external ear
- Pain when eating
- Discharge: often offensive
- Ear canal: swollen, erythematous, exudative, oedematous external auditory canal

Management

- Analgesia: see Section 1.3
- Ear swab for microscopy, culture and sensitivity
- Topical antibiotic eardrops, e.g. gentamycin with hydrocortisone (Gentisone® HC)
- Referral to ENT for micro-suctioning of purulent discharge under microscopy followed by insertion of a gauze wick covered in antibiotic ointment

ACUTE OTITIS MEDIA (AOM)

Definition
- Infection of middle ear
- Common in children
- Frequently bilateral

Aetiology
- *Streptococcus pneumonia*
- *Haemophilus influenza*
- *Moraxella catarrhalis*

Clinical features
- See Table 16.1 and Fig. 16.1
- May become chronic

Table 16.1 **Stages of acute otitis media**

STAGE	CLINICAL FEATURES	MANAGEMENT
Pre-suppurative stage	• Tympanic membrane • Bulging • Intact • Red • Conductive deafness • Otalgia • Fever • Malaise	• Analgesia • Antibiotics if: • No improvement by 48 h • Systemic symptoms present • Cochlear implant • High-risk children • Bilateral AOM
Suppurative stage	• Perforated tympanic membrane • Blood-stained ear discharge • Relief of otalgia	• Swab for culture and sensitivities • Topical antibiotic drops
Acute mastoiditis (can occur due to acute otitis media)	• Erythematous tender mastoid bone with ear pinna protrusion • Unwell • Otalgia • Ear discharge	• Intravenous antibiotics • Analgesia • Refer to ENT

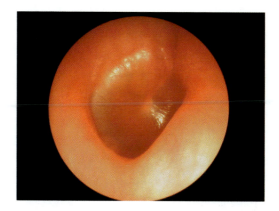

Fig. 16.1 Otitis media. (From Sidwell, R. and Thompson, M., *Easy Paediatrics*, CRC Press, Boca Raton, FL, 2011.)

ACUTE HEARING LOSS

Aetiology

- Viral illness
- Vascular compromise to cochlea
- Intra-cochlear membrane rupture
- Secondary to immune-mediated disease
- Benign positional vertigo
- Labyrinthitis
- Ménière disease
- Syphilis
- Acoustic neuroma
- Cerumen impaction
- Often no cause found

Management

- Refer to ENT once cerumen impaction has been ruled out

16.2 THE NOSE

EPISTAXIS

Aetiology

- Young children and adults:
  - Bleeding often originates from 'Little's area'/'Kiesselbach's area'
  - Area rich in small vessels supplied by internal and external carotid arteries

- Elderly patients:
  - Bleeding originates higher than/posterior to Little's area
  - More difficult to control
- Causes:
  - Trauma
  - Foreign body
  - Bleeding polyp
  - Tumour
  - Coagulopathies
  - Hypertension
  - Idiopathic

Risk factors

- 80% have no predisposing factors
- Warfarin, aspirin, clopidogrel use
- Hypertension

Management

- See Table 16.2

Table 16.2 **Management of epistaxis**

General management	• Resuscitate
	• IV fluids
	• Blood tests:
	  • FBC
	  • G&S and cross-match
	  • Clotting screen
	• Stabilization of any contributing factors
	• See Chapter 9, Haematology, for correction of abnormal clotting

Anterior bleeding	• Mild bleeding:
	  • Sit forward, loosen tight clothing
	  • Encourage patient to blow nose gently to clear clots and to spit out swallowed blood into a disposable receiver dish
	  • Pinch the soft anterior nose to apply pressure over Little's area
	  • Cauterize visible bleeding sources with a silver nitrate stick
	• Moderate to severe bleeding:
	  • Rapid Rhino® or Merocel® tampon nasal packing
	  • BIPP (bismuth iodoform paraffin paste) pack usually inserted by ENT specialists
	  • Admit all patients requiring nasal packing to ENT

(Continued)

Table 16.2 (*Continued*) **Management of epistaxis**

Posterior bleeding	• Posterior-nasal packing • Foley catheter: balloon inflated in post-nasal space to tamponade bleeding or formal posterior nose pack • Anterior BIPP pack usually inserted by ENT specialists • Admit to ENT for close monitoring because of the nasopulmonary reflex which can result in bradydysrhythmias and hypoxia

MICRO-case

An 85-year-old female is brought to the ED. She has been having a nose bleed for the past 40 min that is not stopping. She has had a few minor nose bleeds recently, but they have always stopped within 10 min. She has a past medical history of hypertension and atrial fibrillation for which she is on warfarin.

On examination her heart rate is 110 beats/min, blood pressure is 100/60 mmHg, clotted blood is present in her right nostril but her left nostril is bleeding heavily. Urgent IV access is obtained and blood tests taken. A nasal tampon is inserted into both nostrils. The bleeding appears to cease for 10 min, after which blood starts dripping out from the pack and the patient is also spitting out big blood clots.

The nasal packs are then removed, and a Foley catheter is inserted and inflated into the post-nasal space. Tampons are replaced in both nostrils to stop the bleeding pending formal ENT review and management.

Her haemoglobin result comes back as 8 g/dL and INR 6.

Learning points:

- Epistaxis can be very severe in elderly patients who have more comorbidities. Bleeding is more likely to occur posterior to the Little's area which is often more difficult to control.
- The patient is usually hypertensive and the fact that her BP is 100/60 indicates the severity of the epistaxis.
- This patient will need a blood transfusion and her warfarin will need stopping and reversal with vitamin K, after an urgent discussion with a haematologist. Please refer to Chapter 9, Haematology.
- The patient will need admission under ENT and possible surgical intervention to stop the bleeding.

NASAL FRACTURE

Aetiology

- Usually following direct trauma to the face

Clinical features

- Epistaxis
- Flattening and deformity of the nasal bridge
- Soft tissue swelling

Management

- Check for a septal haematoma:
  - Appears as a cherry red swelling to the nasal septum.
  - Requires urgent incision and drainage by ENT to prevent resulting septal necrosis. Needs antibiotic cover.
- Check airway patency.
- Treat epistaxis.
- Refer to ENT if severe epistaxis or severe nasal deformity.
- Otherwise arrange ENT outpatient review at around 10 days once swelling has subsided to allow for nasal manipulation under anaesthesia should deformity be present.

16.3 THROAT

PHARYNGITIS AND TONSILLITIS

Aetiology

- 70% caused by viruses
- Viral:
  - Adenovirus
  - Rhinoviruses
  - Enteroviruses
  - Influenza virus
  - Parainfluenza virus
  - Epstein-Barr virus (EBV)
- Bacterial:
  - *Streptococcus pyogenes*
  - *Streptococcus pneumoniae*
  - *Haemophilus influenzae*
  - *Mycoplasma pneumoniae*

Clinical features

- Pharyngitis:
  - Sore throat
  - Myalgia
  - Fever
  - Coryzal symptoms

- Tonsillitis:
  - Sore throat
  - Lymphadenopathy
  - Dysphagia
  - Malaise
  - Pyrexia
  - Fever
  - Tonsils:
    - Swollen
    - With or without exudates
- Scarlet fever: *Steptococcus pyogenes* sore throat with an erythematous rash and strawberry red tongue due to toxin production, requiring 10 days of phenoxymethylpenicillin if not allergic

Complications

- Peritonsillar abscess (quinsy)
- Retropharyngeal abscess
- Group A *Streptococcus*:
  - Post-infective rheumatic fever
  - Glomerulonephritis

Management

- Analgesia: see Section 1.3
- Antibiotics for exudative tonsillitis:
  - See NICE Centor criteria in Chapter 14, Paediatrics
  - Penicillin V PO 500 mg QDS for 10 days
- Antiseptic gargles
- Rarely acute tonsillitis can be very severe and require hospital admission:
  - IV fluids
  - IV antibiotics penicillin V 1 g QDS and metronidazole 500 mg TDS
  - IV dexamethasone – if airway compromise

MICRO-facts

Do not give amoxicillin in suspected tonsillitis as this may result in a widespread maculopapular rash if the diagnosis is actually infectious mononucleosis (EBV)!

PERITONSILLAR ABSCESS

Definition

- Abscess between tonsil and pharyngeal muscles
- Also known as a 'quinsy'
- A complication of tonsillitis

Clinical features

- Worsening of symptoms of tonsillitis
- Muffled voice
- Trismus: inability to open mouth
- Dysphagia
- Unilateral swelling of soft palate
- Inflamed tonsils
- Displacement of tonsil downward and medially
- Uvula deviated to unaffected side

Management

- IV fluids
- IV antibiotics:
  - Benzylpenicillin
  - Metronidazole
- IV dexamethasone
- Refer to ENT for incision/aspiration and drainage under local anaesthetic

INFECTIOUS MONONUCLEOSIS

Aetiology

- Epstein-Barr virus (EBV)

> **MICRO-facts**
>
> EBV can cause hepatosplenomegaly and result in these organs being more prone to damage. Contact sports should therefore be avoided for up to 3 months.

Clinical features

- Pyrexia
- Malaise
- Sore throat
- Dysphagia
- Fibrous exudate covering tonsils
- Cervical lymphadenopathy
- Hepatosplenomegaly

> **MICRO-print**
>
> A similar clinical picture may be seen with cytomegalovirus, and toxoplasmosis.

Investigations

- Paul-Bunnell monospot test
- Serum EBV IgM to confirm diagnosis

Management

- Analgesia: see Section 1.3
- Penicillin can be used but not amoxicillin as above
- Avoid close contact with others as virus is infectious for up to 3 months
- Avoid contact sports for 3 months

16.4 FOREIGN BODIES

EAR

- Common in children
- Often quite difficult to remove if poor cooperation from patient
- May need general anaesthetic for removal
- Always check tympanic membrane for perforation after removal

NOSE

- Common in children
- May remain in place for a long time
- Unilateral foul-smelling blood-stained nasal discharge
- Often expelled by asking the carer of the child to perform mother's kiss (see MICRO-print, 'Mother's kiss')
- If unable to remove by suction or gentle instrumentation, requires removal by ENT under general anaesthetic

> **MICRO-print**
> **Mother's kiss**
> A finger is placed over the unaffected nostril; the carer then places his or her mouth over the child's mouth and delivers a short, sharp puff of air. This may dislodge the object through the obstructed nostril.

THROAT

- May occur in adults and children
- Common objects:
  - Coins
  - Toys
  - Food
  - Meat
  - Fish bones
  - Nuts

Emergency and acute medicine

- Presentation:
  - Asymptomatic
  - Cough
  - Shortness of breath
  - Dysphagia/odynophagia
  - Excessive salivation
- Pharynx and oesophagus:
  - Fish bones often impact at the base of the tongue or tonsil.
  - A scratch from a passing foreign body can give a persistent foreign body sensation.
  - Investigation:
    - Visualize posterior pharynx by depressing the tongue.
    - Lateral neck X-ray if radio-opaque object.
  - Refer to the ENT team for further management.
  - Tracheal and bronchial foreign bodies can cause acute airway obstruction necessitating immediate removal by suction, Magill forceps or bronchoscopy. Senior ENT and anaesthetic assistance should be sought.
- Oesophagus:
  - Swallowed objects
  - Lateral neck X-ray and CXR if aspiration suspected
  - Refer to ENT if:
    - Airway obstruction
    - Dangerous object ingested, such as a battery or magnets
  - Discharge if:
    - Asymptomatic
    - X-rays normal
  - Objects will often pass spontaneously
  - Ask patient to return if symptoms develop or the object has not passed

16.5 FACIAL NERVE PALSY

Clinical features

- See Table 16.3

Table 16.3 **Features of facial nerve palsy**

TYPE	FEATURES	CAUSE
Upper motor neurone lesion	• Sparing of upper forehead muscles • Often other neurological signs present	• Cerebrovascular accident

(Continued)

Table 16.3 *(Continued)* **Features of facial nerve palsy**

TYPE	FEATURES	CAUSE
Lower motor neurone lesion	• Involvement of whole side of face and forehead	• Bell's palsy • Ramsay Hunt syndrome • Trauma • Tumour

BELL'S PALSY

Aetiology

- Thought to be virally induced

Clinical features

- Postauricular pain
- Hyperacusis: certain frequencies of sound seem abnormally loud
- Abnormal taste in the anterior two-thirds of tongue

Management

- Course of high-dose steroids, e.g. prednisolone 60 mg once daily for 5 to 7 days. Oral aciclovir may also be used according to local ENT preference.
- Diligent eye care – eye drops/eye patch to prevent corneal ulceration.
- ENT follow-up.

RAMSAY HUNT SYNDROME

Aetiology

- Varicella zoster virus (VZV)
- Infecting geniculate ganglion
- With or without involvement of the facial nerve

Clinical features

- Vesicles present in external ear canal

Management

- Antiviral: aciclovir – shortens duration of palsy
- Steroids may be considered – consult local guidelines

MICRO-print

House-Brackmann grading system for facial palsy

Used by ENT specialists to classify facial palsy.

I	No weakness
II	Slight weakness
	Complete eye closure
	Normal forehead movement
	Mouth slightly weak
III	Complete eye closure with effort
	Moderate forehead movement
	Mouth slightly weak
IV	Obvious asymmetry between both sides of face
	No forehead movement
	Incomplete eye closure
V	Asymmetrical at rest
	No forehead movements
	Incomplete eye closure
	Slight mouth movement
VI	No movement

16.6 VERTIGO

Clinical features

- See Table 16.4

Table 16.4 **Causes of vertigo**

	PERIPHERAL CAUSES	CENTRAL CAUSES
Features	• More common • Lesion in vestibular nerve and inner ear	• Less common • Lesion in central nervous system

(Continued)

Table 16.4 *(Continued)* **Causes of vertigo**

	PERIPHERAL CAUSES	CENTRAL CAUSES
Causes	• Acute labyrinthitis • Menière's disease • Benign positional vertigo • Otitis media • Trauma • Secondary to ototoxic drugs	• Stroke • TIA • Cerebellopontine angle tumour
Clinical features	• Deafness • Nausea and vomiting • Nystagmus	• Cranial nerve deficits • Vertical nystagmus • Ataxia
Management	• Manage cause • Central causes should be referred to the medical team for further investigation • Prochlorperazine 12.5 mg IM	

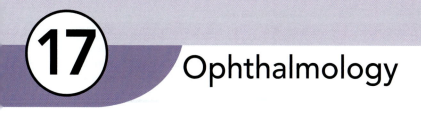

17 Ophthalmology

17.1 THE ACUTELY RED EYE

Causes

- See Table 17.1

Table 17.1 **Causes of red eye**

CONDITION	AETIOLOGY	CLINICAL FEATURES	MANAGEMENT

Acute conjunctivitis	• Allergic
	• Bacterial
	  • *Staphylococci*
	  • *Pneumococcus*
	  • *Haemophilus*
	  • *Neisseria gonorrhoea*
	• Viral: adenovirus
		• Red, inflamed conjunctiva
		• Sticky discharge
		• Gritty discomfort
			• Sodium cromoglicate drops if allergic
			• Antibiotic eye drops/ointment for 5 days: chloramphenicol
			• Advise not to share towels/good hygiene
			• Avoid cosmetics to eye

Episcleritis	• May be sectorial	• Dull ache • Red eye	• Oral NSAIDs • Refer to ophthalmology
Scleritis	• Systemic lupus erythematous • Rheumatoid arthritis	• Painful • Diffusely red • Sore	• Oral NSAIDs • Refer to ophthalmology–steroid eye drops
Acute iritis (anterior uveitis)	• Idiopathic • Ulcerative colitis • Crohn's disease • Ankylosing spondylitis	• Painful, tender eye • Reduced visual acuity • Small pupil • Circumcorneal erythema • Pus present in anterior chamber	• Urgent ophthalmology referral • Steroid eye drops • Analgesia: see Section 1.3

(Continued)

Table 17.1 *(Continued)* **Causes of red eye**

CONDITION	AETIOLOGY	CLINICAL FEATURES	MANAGEMENT
Acute keratitis	• Contact lens use • Herpes simplex virus • Bacterial infection	• Severe pain • Fluorescein staining of eye may show corneal ulceration on slit lamp examination	• Urgent ophthalmology referral
Acute closed-angle glaucoma	• Raised intraocular pressure • Narrow anterior chamber • Sudden obstruction to outflow of aqueous humour	• Severe, intense eye pain • Headache • Nausea/vomiting • Reduced visual acuity • Fixed, semi-dilated ovoid pupil • Ciliary flush with hazy cornea	• Urgent ophthalmology review • Analgesia: see Section 1.3 • Antiemetic, e.g. metoclopramide 10 mg • Miotic drops– pilocarpine or β-blocker eye drops, e.g. timolol • IV or oral acetazolamide

17.2 ACUTE VISUAL LOSS

Causes

• See Table 17.2

Table 17.2 **Causes of vision loss**

CONDITION	AETIOLOGY	CLINICAL FEATURES	MANAGEMENT

Central retinal artery occlusion		• Sudden painless loss of vision
		• Direct pupil reaction is slow/absent
		• Responds to consensual stimulation
		• Fundoscopy reveals:
		  • Pale optic disc
		  • Cherry red spot at macula
			• Urgent ophthalmology review
			• Reduce intra-ocular pressure:
			  • IV or oral acetozolamide
			  • Digitally massage eye for 5 s every 10 s
			• Rule out temporal arteritis

(Continued)

Table 17.2 *(Continued)* **Causes of vision loss**

CONDITION	AETIOLOGY	CLINICAL FEATURES	MANAGEMENT

Central retinal vein occlusion	• Atheromatous disease
	• Chronic glaucoma
		• Sudden painless loss of vision
		• Direct pupil reaction is slow/absent
		• Responds to consensual stimulation
		• Fundoscopy reveals: Optic disc swelling
		  • Congested veins
		  • Flame-shaped haemorrhages
			• Ophthalmology review to prevent other eye being affected

Retinal detachment	• Occurs spontaneously in:
	  • Elderly
	  • Diabetics
	  • Myopic patients
	• May occur following trauma or vitreous haemorrhage
		• History of floaters and sudden flashes of light
		• Peripheral visual loss which is profound if macula is affected
		• Fundoscopy reveals dark opaque retina
			• Immediate ophthalmology review
			• Possible surgical repair

Temporal arteritis (giant cell arteritis)	• Inflammation of posterior ciliary arteries • Associated with polymyalgia rheumatica • Refer to neurology; see 'Headache' section in Chapter 6	• Headaches • Malaise • Muscle aches • Jaw claudication pain • Tender temporal arteries • Raised ESR • Fundoscopy reveals pale optic disc	• IV or oral steroids • Urgent ophthalmology review

(Continued)

Emergency and acute medicine

Table 17.2 *(Continued)* **Causes of vision loss**

CONDITION	AETIOLOGY	CLINICAL FEATURES	MANAGEMENT
Optic neuritis	• Optic nerve inflammation • Associated with multiple sclerosis	• Gradual visual loss • Internuclear ophthalmoplegia • Reduced colour vision • Fundoscopy reveals a swollen optic disc	• Ophthalmology referral • Often recover untreated • May need steroids

17.3 ORBITAL CELLULITIS

Aetiology

- Often a complication of acute sinusitis or post-sinus surgery
- Following periorbital injury

Clinical features (Table 17.3 and Fig. 17.1)

- Fever
- Eyelid swelling
- Congested eye
- Ophthalmoplegia
- Reduced painful eye movements
- Exopthalmos

Table 17.3 **Differences between pre-septal and post-septal cellulitis**

CONDITION	CLINICAL FEATURES	MANAGEMENT
Pre-septal (periorbital) cellulitis	• Periocular superficial cellulitis • Less serious • No/minimal systemic upset • Eye is not involved	• Oral or IV antibiotics depending on severity • May need admission

Post-septal (orbital cellulitis)	• Orbital deep cellulitis
	• Serious
	• Systemic upset
	• Involvement of eye
	  • Inflamed sclera/conjunctiva
	  • Painful eye movements
	  • Diplopia
	  • Impaired acuity and colour vision
		• IV antibiotics and admission

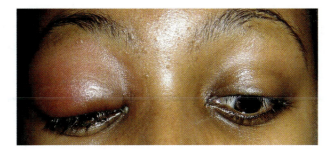

Fig. 17.1 Pre-septal cellulitis and orbital cellulitis. (From Sidwell, R. and Thompson, M., *Easy Paediatrics*, CRC Press, Boca Raton, FL, 2011.)

Management

- Blood tests:
  - FBC
  - CRP
  - Blood cultures
- IV antibiotics: cefotaxime IV 1 g QDS
- Immediate referral to ophthalmology and ENT
- CT scan

17.4 FOREIGN BODY (FB)

Aetiology

- Often grit that has blown into the eye
- Metal from industrial source

Clinical features

- Red, watering eye
- Painful to blink
- FB sensation

Examination

- Instill local anaesthetic eye drops
- Use slit lamp to examine eye
- Evert upper and lower eyelids to check for subtarsal foreign bodies

Management

- Conjunctival foreign body:
  - Use moist cotton bud to remove.

- Corneal foreign body:
    - Use moist cotton bud to remove.
    - If difficult to remove, use bevel end of hypodermic needle; instill fluorescein to check for corneal abrasion.
    - Chloramphenicol eye drops or ointment for 5 days.
    - Consider outpatient ophthalmology review.

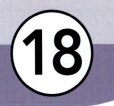

Infectious diseases

18.1 NOTIFIABLE DISEASES

Definition
- A list of diseases, cases of which the local health authority must be notified

MICRO-facts

- Acute encephalitis
- Acute meningitis
- Acute poliomyelitis
- Acute infectious hepatitis
- Anthrax
- Botulism
- Brucellosis
- Cholera
- Diphtheria
- Enteric fever (typhoid or paratyphoid)
- Food poisoning
- Haemolytic uraemic syndrome (HUS)
- Infectious bloody diarrhoea
- Invasive Group A streptococcal disease and scarlet fever
- Legionnaire disease
- Leprosy
- Malaria
- Measles
- Meningococcal septicaemia
- Mumps
- Plague
- Rabies
- Rubella
- SARS
- Smallpox
- Tetanus
- Tuberculosis
- Typhus

continued...

continued...
- Viral haemorrhagic fever
- Whooping cough
- Yellow fever

It is the duty of the attending doctor to notify the local health authority of both diagnosis and clinical suspicion of any of the above.

18.2 EMPIRICAL ANTIBIOTIC DOSES

- These are to be used as a guideline for the first-line treatment of common infections (Table 18.1).
- Always consult local guidelines.
- Antibiotics may need to be reviewed once MC&S result is known.

Table 18.1 **Empirical antibiotic doses for common infections**

INFECTION	FIRST-LINE TREATMENT	COMMENTS
Non-severe community-acquired pneumonia	• Amoxicillin (PO) 500 mg 8 hourly • (Penicillin allergy) Clarithromycin (PO) 500 mg 12 hourly	• Only add clarithromycin if an atypical pathogen is likely • Atypical pneumonia unlikely in patients >65 (1%) • See Pneumonia, Section 4.5
Severe community-acquired pneumonia	• Amoxicillin (IV) 1 g 8 hourly + clarithromycin (IV) 500 mg 12 hourly	• Labs often suggest switching IV to oral clarithromycin after 48 h
Aspiration pneumonia	• Co-amoxiclav (IV) 1.2 g 8 hourly • Total duration 5 days (IV + PO)	• Switch to oral as soon as condition permits
Exacerbation of chronic bronchitis	• Community acquired: • Amoxicillin (PO) 500 mg 8 hourly for 5 days • (Penicillin allergy) Doxycycline (PO) 200 mg on day 1, then 100 mg once daily for 5 days	• Hospital acquired: • Co-amoxiclav (PO) 625 mg 8 hourly for 5 days

(Continued)

Table 18.1 *(Continued)* **Empirical antibiotic doses for common infections**

INFECTION	FIRST-LINE TREATMENT	COMMENTS

Cellulitis	• Severe (IV):
	  • Benzylpenicillin 1.2 g 4 hourly
	  • + Flucloxacillin 1 g 6 hourly
	  • (Penicillin allergy) Clindamycin (PO) 450 mg 6 hourly
		• Mild (oral):
		  • Amoxicillin 500 mg 8 hourly
		  • + Flucloxacillin 500 mg 6 hourly
		  • (Penicillin allergy) Clindamycin (PO) 450 mg 6 hourly

Meningitis	• Cefotaxime (IV) 2 g 6 hourly
	• If >55 years old, add amoxicillin (IV) 2 g 4 hourly to cover *Listeria*
		• Contact microbiology/ ID if:
		  • Immunocompromised
		  • Post-neurosurgery
		  • Suspected abscess

C. difficile diarrhoea	• Metronidazole (PO) 400 mg 8 hourly • Vancomycin (PO) second line	• Treat for 14 days

Urinary tract infection	• Trimethoprim (PO) 200 mg 12 hourly
	• Second line (if above has already failed):
	  • Nitrofurantoin (PO) 50 mg 6 hourly
	  • Co-amoxiclav (PO) 375 mg 8 hourly
	• Severe: co-amoxiclav 625 mg 8 hourly or contact microbiologist
		• 3 days should be adequate if uncomplicated
		• Long-term catheterization often results in bacteriuria; avoid antibiotics unless systemically unwell
		• Trimethoprim – avoid in the first trimester of pregnancy and significant renal impairment
		• Nitrofurantoin – avoid in renal impairment

Biliary tract infection	• Co-amoxiclav (IV) 1.2 g 8 hourly	• (Penicillin allergy) Contact microbiology

(Continued)

Table 18.1 *(Continued)* **Empirical antibiotic doses for common infections**

INFECTION	FIRST-LINE TREATMENT	COMMENTS

Abdominal infection	• <65 years old:
	  • Cefuroxime (IV) 750–1500 mg 8 hourly
	  • + Metronidazole (IV) 500 mg 8 hourly
		• >65 years old:
		  • Piperacillin/tazobactam (IV) 4.5 g 8 hourly

Acute osteomyelitis/ septic arthritis	• Flucloxacillin (IV) 1 g 6 hourly • + Sodium fusidate (PO) 500 mg 8 hourly	• (Penicillin allergy) Discuss with microbiology • Prolonged treatment required

Contact microbiology	• In cases of:
	  • Hospital-acquired pneumonia endocarditis
	  • Septicaemia of unknown origin
	  • MRSA infection
		• For advice:
		  • In penicillin allergy
		  • If unsure

> **MICRO-reference**
> Based on Sheffield Teaching Hospitals Trust guidelines.

18.3 GASTROENTERITIS

Definition

- Infection of the stomach and bowel

> **MICRO-facts**
> Gastroenteritis is common. One in five people in England is affected every year.

Risk factors

- Faeco-oral transmission:
  - Food poisoning/contact with contaminated objects
  - Close contact with other affected persons
  - Recent travel abroad
- Recent antibiotics, chemotherapy (*Clostridium difficile*)

Clinical features

- Diarrhoea (≥3 episodes within a 24 h period)
- ± Vomiting
- Abdominal pain/cramps
- Fever
- Dehydration

> ## MICRO-facts
>
> - Keep in mind more serious causes of diarrhoea, such as bowel cancer.
> - Thorough history taking is vital.

Investigations

- Stool sample: MC&S (if recent travel or antibiotics, food handler or severely ill)

Management

- See Fig. 18.1

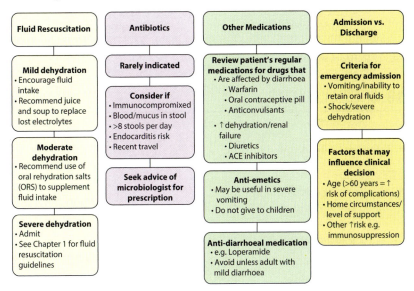

Fig. 18.1 Management of gastroenteritis.

Transmission avoidance

- Patients should:
  - Wash their hands regularly
  - Avoid food preparation
  - Not return to work until 48 h after their last episode of diarrhoea

Complications

- Toxic megacolon:
    - Complication of *C. difficile* infection
    - Inflammation spreads to the smooth muscle layer of the bowel
    - Presents with abdominal pain and shock
    - Perform abdominal X-ray
    - Contact surgical team for advice ± review
- Haemolytic uraemic syndrome:
    - A rare complication of *E. coli* O157:H7 infection
    - Avoid antibiotics
    - May require dialysis
    - Presents with the triad of symptoms: shown in Fig. 18.2

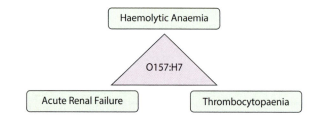

Fig. 18.2 Haemolytic uraemic syndrome.

18.4 CELLULITIS

Definition

- Infection of the dermis

Aetiology

- Skin flora organisms:
    - *Staphylococcus aureus*
    - *Streptococcus pyogenes*
    - *Pseudomonas* spp.

Risk factors

- Diabetes mellitus
- Other causes of immunocompromise, e.g. HIV, chemotherapy
- IV drug use
- Source of infection, e.g. foreign body, trauma, cracked skin

Clinical features

- General:
    - Erythema with poorly defined margins
    - Warmth, pain and swelling

- Systemic:
  - Fever, chills and malaise
  - Regional lymphadenopathy
  - Ascending lymphangitis (red streaking of skin around infection)

Investigations
- Bloods: FBC, blood cultures
- MC&S: swab of wound
- X-ray:
  - Bone invasion (osteomyelitis)
  - Gas in soft tissues (may require surgery)
  - Foreign body
- Venous Doppler to exclude DVT

Management
- Outline margins
- Immobilize and elevate the affected region
- Analgesia
- Antibiotics (see Fig. 18.3)

MICRO-facts

Monitor the progression/treatment of all soft tissue infections:
- Draw around the margin of the infected area.
- Mark the date and time at which the line was drawn.
- A rapidly spreading infection may be fatal if not recognized.

18.5 ERYSIPELAS

Definition
- Acute skin infection of the epidermis (more superficial than cellulitis)

Aetiology
- *S. pyogenes* (Group A β-haemolytic *Streptococcus*)

Clinical features
- Erythema with a sharp line of demarcation
- Induration (thickening/hardening) of infected skin

MICRO-facts

Cellulitis vs. erysipelas
- Cellulitis = poorly defined margins
- Erysipelas = sharply defined margins

Management

- Antibiotics (see Fig. 18.3)

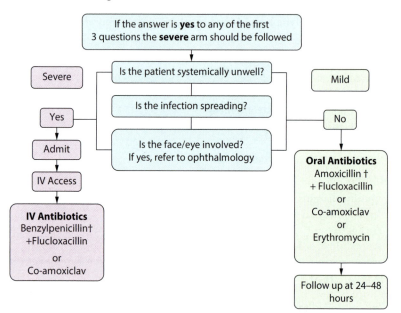

Fig. 18.3 Antibiotic treatment of cellulitis and erysipelas.

18.6 NECROTIZING FASCIITIS

Definition

- Rapidly spreading necrotic infection of the deep fascia

> **MICRO-facts**
>
> Necrotizing fasciitis can lead to loss of limb and death and so must be recognized and treated quickly.

Aetiology

- Type I: β-haemolytic *Streptococcus*
- Type II: polymicrobial

Clinical features

- Severe pain (may be out of proportion to the other clinical symptoms)
- Fever

- Oedema
- Crepitus (subcutaneous gas)
- Patient appears toxic
- Skin becomes blue/black (necrosis) and blistered

> **MICRO-print**
> **Fournier's gangrene** is a similar infection involving the abdomen, perineum and scrotum.

Investigations

- Usually a clinical diagnosis
- X-ray shows subcutaneous gas
- Raised creatinine kinase suggests muscle involvement (myonecrosis)

Management

- Aggressive fluid resuscitation
- IV antibiotics (see Fig. 14.3)
- Surgical debridement of affected tissues

> **MICRO-case**
> You are called to the minor injuries department to see a 40-year-old-man with a painful right leg. He has a low-grade fever, and his leg is red, swollen and hot to the touch. The other leg is completely normal. You examine his leg but cannot see any breaks in the skin. The area of redness has indistinct borders, which you draw around, marking on the time. When you return, the redness has not extended past the line. Blood tests show a raised white cell count. You diagnose cellulitis and start a course of oral flucloxacillin and amoxicillin.
> **Key points:**
> - The point of entry of infection may not be visible and is not diagnostic of cellulitis.
> - Those systemically well may be treated as outpatients using oral antibiotics.
> - A swab of the infected area is not required unless the patient is unwell or not responding to antibiotics.
> - A faster-spreading area of redness would prompt concern of necrotizing fasciitis.
> - DVT would be a differential here, with the raised white cell count and clinical appearance making cellulitis the most likely diagnosis.

Emergency and acute medicine

18.7 MENINGITIS AND MENINGOCOCCAL SEPTICAEMIA

For paediatric infection, see Chapter 14.

Definitions

- Meningitis: inflammation of the meningeal tissues that surround the brain
- Meningococcal septicaemia: sepsis caused by *Neisseria meningitidis*

Risk factors

- Parameningeal infection:
  - Otitis media
  - Sinusitis
- Penetrating head trauma
- Immunodeficiency
- Recent neurosurgery e.g. shunt insertion

Aetiology

- Viral 'aseptic':
  - Enteroviruses (account for >80%)
  - Varicella zoster virus (VZV)
  - Herpes simplex virus (HSV) 1 and 2
- Bacterial:
  - Varies with age
  - Adolescents/adults: *Streptococcus pneumoniae, N. meningitidis*
  - Elderly: *S. pneumoniae, N. meningitidis, Listeria monocytogenes*

Clinical features

- See Table 18.2

Table 18.2 **Clinical features of adult meningitis**

CLINICAL FEATURES OF MENINGITIS IN ADULTS	
Symptoms	• Headache • Nausea and vomiting • Neck stiffness • Lethargy

(Continued)

Table 18.2 (Continued) **Clinical features of adult meningitis**

CLINICAL FEATURES OF MENINGITIS IN ADULTS	

Signs	• Fever
	• Altered consciousness
	• Seizures
	• Signs of meningeal inflammation:
	  • Brudzinski's sign: passive neck flexion causes bilateral hip/knee flexion
	  • Kernig's sign: knee extension causes pain/resistance to movement
	• Signs of meningococcaemia:
	  • Sepsis/shock
	  • Petechial/purpuric rash (late)

Management

- Emergency management: see Fig. 18.4

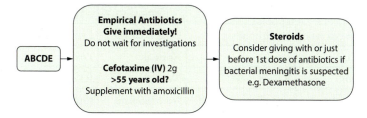

Fig. 18.4 Management of adult meningitis.

Investigations

- Bloods:
    - FBC
    - U&E
    - Glucose
    - LFT
    - CRP
    - Clotting screen
    - Blood gases (ABG)
- Microbiology:
    - Blood cultures (take prior to commencing antibiotics, provided no significant delay)
    - Throat swab
    - Blood for PCR for common pathogens, e.g. meningococcus

Emergency and acute medicine

- CT scan:
  - Rule out sub-arachnoid haemorrhage
  - If focal neurological signs, reduced consciousness, or features of raised intracranial pressure
- Lumbar puncture (LP):
  - Perform fundoscopy to rule out raised intracranial pressure: look for papilloedema
  - Send CSF samples for:
    - Gram stain and microscopy
    - Culture and sensitivity
    - PCR and serology: viral, meningococcal, pneumococcal
    - Glucose (take blood glucose concurrently)
    - Protein

Further management

- Review LP results (see Table 18.3)

Table 18.3 **Differential lumbar puncture results for infective meningitis**

	BACTERIAL	VIRAL	TUBERCULOSIS
White cell type	Neutrophils	Lymphocytes	Lymphocytes
Glucose	Low	Normal	Low
Protein	Raised	Normal	Raised
Microscopy	Organisms may be visible on gram stain	No organisms visible	Organisms may be visible on Ziehl-Neelson staining
Further tests	Culture Meningococcal and pneumococcal PCR	Viral PCR for enterovirus, VZV, HSV	TB culture

- Adjust antibiotics according to results of gram stain/MC&S
- Continue dexamethasone for 4 days
- Notify the Health Protection Agency (HPA)
- Contact prophylaxis if *N. meningitidis*:
  - Rifampicin
  - Ciprofloxacin 500 mg stat

MICRO-print

If features of encephalitis are present, e.g. altered consciousness, abnormal behaviour, focal neurology, seizures, treat with aciclovir in addition to antibiotics.

18.8 INFECTIVE ENDOCARDITIS

Definition
- Infection of cardiac endothelium

Risk factors
- High-risk physiology:
  - Prosthetic heart valve
  - Previous infective endocarditis
  - Unrepaired congenital heart disease
- Moderate-risk physiology:
  - Valvular dysfunction
  - Other congenital heart disease
- Increased risk of bacteraemia:
  - Intravenous drug use
  - Dental caries
  - Indwelling venous catheter, e.g. central venous pressure line

> ## MICRO-facts
>
> All patients with a fever and new or changing murmur should be investigated for infective endocarditis.

Clinical features
- See Table 18.4

Table 18.4 **Features of infective endocarditis**

	FEATURES
Systemic	• Fever • Rigors • Night sweats • Weight loss
Cardiac	• Chest pain • Dyspnoea • Clubbing • New/exacerbated regurgitant murmur • Heart failure

(Continued)

Emergency and acute medicine

Table 18.4 *(Continued)* **Features of infective endocarditis**

	FEATURES
Vascular	• Splinter haemorrhages • Janeway lesions: painless red macules on palms • Focal neurological signs – suggestive of a thrombotic event • Splenomegaly • Microscopic haematuria
Immune	• Osler's nodes: painful, red, raised lesions on fingers • Glomerulonephritis • Arthritis • Roth's spots: retinal haemorrhages with blanched centres

---

MICRO-print

Incidence of valve involvement

Mitral > Aortic > Tricuspid > Pulmonary

Investigations
- Bloods:
    - FBC: anaemia (normochromic, normocytic)
    - ESR: ↑
    - Rheumatoid factor: +ve
    - Serial blood cultures:
        - 3 sets over 24 h period
        - Different sites
        - >1 h apart
- Urinalysis: proteinuria
- ECG: ↑ PR interval may indicate perivalvular abscess

Diagnosis
- Duke's modified criteria (Fig. 18.5)

Management
- Admit for investigation/treatment:
    - Cardiology
    - Infectious diseases

Further investigation
- Echocardiogram
    - Transthoracic echo (TTE):
        - May be used as initial investigation
        - Negative result does not exclude endocarditis

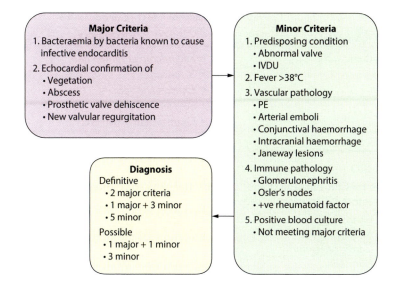

Major Criteria
1. Bacteraemia by bacteria known to cause infective endocarditis
2. Echocardial confirmation of
   • Vegetation
   • Abscess
   • Prosthetic valve dehiscence
   • New valvular regurgitation

Minor Criteria
1. Predisposing condition
   • Abnormal valve
   • IVDU
2. Fever >38°C
3. Vascular pathology
   • PE
   • Arterial emboli
   • Conjunctival haemorrhage
   • Intracranial haemorrhage
   • Janeway lesions
4. Immune pathology
   • Glomerulonephritis
   • Osler's nodes
   • +ve rheumatoid factor
5. Positive blood culture
   • Not meeting major criteria

Diagnosis
Definitive
   • 2 major criteria
   • 1 major + 3 minor
   • 5 minor
Possible
   • 1 major + 1 minor
   • 3 minor

Fig. 18.5 Diagnostic criteria for infective endocarditis.

- Trans-oesophageal echo (TOE):
  - Definitive investigation
  - Assess for:
    ○ Vegetation
    ○ Abscess
    ○ Regurgitation

Aetiology

- See Table 18.5

Table 18.5 **Causative organisms of infective endocarditis**

EPIDEMIOLOGY	ORGANISM
Native valve	• *Streptococcus* spp. • *S. aureus* • Enterococcus • Gram-negative bacteria
IVDU	• *S. aureus* • Enterococcus • Gram-negative bacteria • *Candida* spp.

(Continued)

Table 18.5 *(Continued)* **Causative organisms of infective endocarditis**

EPIDEMIOLOGY	ORGANISM
Prosthetic valve	• *Staphylococcus epidermidis* • *S. aureus* • *Enterococcus* spp. • *Streptococcus* spp. • Gram-negative bacteria

---

MICRO-print

The **HACEK** bacteria do not grow on standard agar. Their culture must therefore be specifically requested.

- *Haemophilus*
- *Actinobacillus*
- *Cardiobacterium*
- *Eikenella*
- *Kingella*

Treatment

- Antibiotics:
  - Consult microbiology and treat according to culture/sensitivity
  - See Table 18.6
  - Always consult local guidelines

Table 18.6 **Treatment of infective endocarditis**

CIRCUMSTANCES	ANTIBIOTIC
Empirical	• Flucloxacillin + benzylpenicillin • Gentamicin
Empirical, with cardiac prostheses	• Rifampicin + vancomycin
Staphylococci	• Flucloxacillin • Rifampicin + vancomycin (if MRSA/penicillin allergy)
Streptococci	• Benzylpenicillin + gentamicin • Vancomycin + gentamicin (if penicillin allergy/resistance)
Enterococci	• Amoxicillin + gentamicin • Vancomycin + gentamicin (if penicillin allergy/resistance)

(Continued)

Emergency and acute medicine

Table 18.6 *(Continued)* **Treatment of infective endocarditis**

CIRCUMSTANCES	ANTIBIOTIC
HACEK organisms	• Amoxicillin + gentamicin • Ceftriaxone + gentamicin (if penicillin allergy/resistance)
Fungi	• Amphotericin • Fluconazole • Flucytosine

- Surgical:
    - Consider prosthetic valves if:
        - Severe damage to native valves
        - Infected prostheses

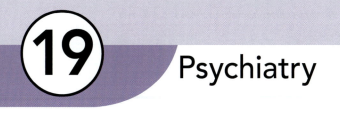

19 Psychiatry

19.1 DELIBERATE SELF-HARM

Causes
- Psychiatric disorder
- Physical disorder
- Substance misuse/dependence/withdrawal
- Acute and chronic life stresses:
  - Relationships
  - Financial
  - Housing
  - Employment/studies
  - Social isolation

Methods of self-harm
- Medication overdose: e.g. paracetamol, tricyclic antidepressants, insulin
- Illicit drug overdose: e.g. opioids, cocaine
- Physical injury: wrist cutting, hanging

> **MICRO-facts**
>
> Actively suicidal patients must not leave hospital without a psychiatry assessment.

Assessing suicidal intent
- Premeditated and careful preparation
- Organized will, final acts
- Carrying out act alone with no intention of being found
- Violent method
- Not seeking help following self-harm
- Continuing suicidal ideation and intent

Use SAD Persons Scale as a risk stratification tool (see Table 19.1).

Table 19.1 **SAD Persons scoring system to assess suicide risk**

SAD PERSONS SCALE	SCORE
Sex: Male	1
Age <19 or >45 years	1
Depression	2
Previous suicidal attempt	1
Excessive alcohol/drug use	1
Rational thinking loss	2
Separated, widowed or divorced	1
Organized or serious attempt	2
No social support	1
Stated future intent	2

- Interpreting score:
  - <6: May be safe to discharge
  - 6–8: Recommended psychiatric assessment
  - >8: Admit for urgent psychiatric assessment

Investigations

- Physical examination: full systemic examination
- Psychiatric history and mental state examination:
  - Assess suicide risk
    - Intent at time of act
    - Previous self-harm
    - Ongoing suicidal risk
- Blood tests:
  - LFTs and clotting screen: may be deranged in paracetamol overdose
  - Serum drug levels: paracetamol, salicylate, ethanol
- Urine tests: urine toxicology screen

MICRO-facts

Mental state examination

- Appearance
- Behaviour
- Speech – rate, rhythm, volume, tone
- Mood – objective and subjective
- Thoughts – thought disorder, flight of ideas, knight's move thinking, loosening of association, perseveration, thought block, thought

continued…

continued...

> insertion, withdrawal, broadcasting, abnormal beliefs, delusional perception, overvalued ideas, paranoid ideation
> - Perception – hallucinations
> - Cognition – MMSE
> - Insight

Management

- Minimize further physical harm from act and provide supportive medical care.
- Detect any underlying psychiatric disorder.
- Explore recent stresses and coping resources.
- Admit patient: gives patient opportunity to escape from the source for their self-harm and chance to discuss plans for future.
- Plan for follow up on discharge: psychiatric referral, psychotherapy.

19.2 AGGRESSIVE BEHAVIOUR

Causes

- Acute delirium
- Dementia
- Drug/alcohol intoxication
- Psychosis
- Anger
- Pain

Management

- Assess safety: are you at risk?
- Call for help: staff/security/police
- Sedation if risk to themselves or others:
    - Oral or IM lorazepam 2 mg
    - Oral or IM haloperidol (IV only in exceptional circumstances)
- Attempt to diffuse situation if safe:
    - Listen to patient
    - Address concerns
    - Apologize/offer sympathy
    - If above fails, call for senior help
- Offer oral sedation or analgesia
- When patient has settled, investigate for an underlying cause

> **MICRO-facts**
>
> If a patient is at risk to him/herself or others, the minimum necessary restraint and emergency sedation may be applied without consent under common law.

19.3 SIDE EFFECTS OF ANTIPSYCHOTICS

Clinical features

- Anticholinergic:
  - Dry mouth
  - Blurred vision
  - Urinary retention
  - Constipation
- Sedative
- Extrapyramidal:
  - Drug-induced Parkinsonian signs/symptoms
  - Acute dystonia
  - Akathesia

ACUTE DYSTONIA

Clinical features

- Due to increased muscle tone
  - Head and neck: torticollis
  - Extraocular muscles: oculogyric crisis (eyes roll upwards)
  - Respiratory muscles involved: emergency

Management

- ABC (respiratory support)
- IV procyclidine 5 mg twice daily (5–10 mg as a stat dose)
- PRN procyclidine 20 mg IM or oral

NEUROLEPTIC MALIGNANT SYNDROME

Definition

- Rare hyper-metabolic reaction to dopamine antagonists
- Dopamine receptors are blocked leading to autonomic dysfunction
- Mortality is 10–20%

Aetiology

- Young patients prescribed antipsychotic medication
- Idiosyncratic but occurs if otherwise unwell, e.g. sepsis

Clinical features

- Autonomic instability
- BP: ↑/↓
- Hyperpyrexia
- Sweating
- Dehydration
- Rigidity and posturing: increased muscle tone
- Rhabdomyolysis/thromboembolic phenomena due to severe muscle rigidity

Investigations

- Bloods: ↑ CK, ↑ WCC

Management

- May need urgent transfer to ICU
    - ABCDE: respiratory support
    - Continuous BP check and control
    - ↓ Temperature with conservative measures; may need dantrolene
    - Stop antipsychotic drugs
    - Diazepam: decrease muscle tension
    - Bromocriptine: dopamine agonist

> **MICRO-print**
> Reintroduction of an antipsychotic drug re-triggers the syndrome in up to one-third of patients.

19.4 LITHIUM TOXICITY

Clinical features

- See Table 19.2

> **MICRO-facts**
> Lithium toxicity is a feature of chronic use rather than acute ingestion, which is rarely harmful.
> **Beware: NSAIDs may exacerbate lithium toxicity.**

Table 19.2 **Clinical features of lithium toxicity according to blood levels**

LITHIUM BLOOD LEVELS	CLINICAL FEATURES	MANAGEMENT
1.0–1.5 mmol/L	• Thirst • Dry mouth • Urinary frequency • Fine tremor • Poor concentration • Oedema	• Reassure • Check lithium levels • Check U&Es and TFTs • Continue medication • Educate about toxicity • Psych follow-up to consider change to meds
>1.5 mmol/L	• Coarse tremor • Agitation • Nystagmus • Disorientation • Polyuria • Nausea and vomiting	• Admit patient • Stop lithium • IV fluids • Monitor U&Es • Watch for relapse of bipolar symptoms • Psychiatry team to review medication

>2.0 mmol/L	• Spasms
	• Coma
	• Seizures
	• Arrhythmias
	• Renal failure
		• Urgent admission
		• ABC resuscitation
		• Continuous ECG monitoring
		• Stop lithium
		• Monitor:
		  • Lithium level
		  • U&Es
		  • TFTs
		• IV access and fluids

Emergency and acute medicine

19.5 ALCOHOL ABUSE

CONSEQUENCES OF ALCOHOL ABUSE

- See Fig. 19.1

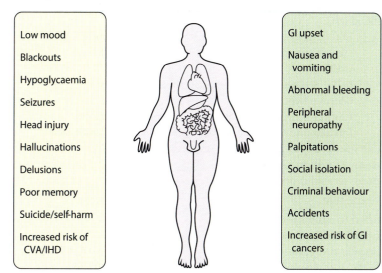

Low mood

Blackouts

Hypoglycaemia

Seizures

Head injury

Hallucinations

Delusions

Poor memory

Suicide/self-harm

Increased risk of CVA/IHD

GI upset

Nausea and vomiting

Abnormal bleeding

Peripheral neuropathy

Palpitations

Social isolation

Criminal behaviour

Accidents

Increased risk of GI cancers

Fig. 19.1 Consequences of alcohol abuse.

ACUTE ALCOHOL TOXICITY

Clinical features

- Slurred/incoherent speech
- Poor coordination
- Unsteady gait
- Vomiting
- Confusion
- Aggression
- Hypoglycaemia
- Injury e.g. head injury
- Coma

Differential diagnosis

- Head injury
- Metabolic disturbance: hypoglycaemia
- Postictal confusion
- Meningitis

Emergency and acute medicine

- Encephalitis
- Drug abuse

Investigations

- Baseline observations: pulse, BP, SpO_2, RR (respiratory depression), ECG (atrial fibrillation, arrhythmias), GCS (may require airway support if lowered)
- Blood tests:
  - FBC: macrocytic anaemia if chronic alcoholism; normal WCC may exclude sepsis as differential
  - U&Es
  - LFTs: deranged transaminases in chronic alcoholism
  - Glucose: hypoglycaemia
  - Clotting screen: may be deranged if hepatic impairment
  - Inflammatory markers: raised in infection and inflammation
- Consider CT head if head injury suspected
- Consider urine toxicology screen
- Assess alcohol dependence

Management

- ABCDE resuscitation
- Close baseline observations
- Regular BM glucose monitoring
- IV fluids if repeated episodes of vomiting
- Treat complications accordingly e.g. head injury and GI bleed (see relevant chapters)
- Coma:
  - ABCDE with C-spine control
  - Recovery position in case of vomiting; exclude causes in differential diagnoses: CT scan and blood glucose
  - Continuous baseline observations
- Discharge if:
  - Conscious
  - Uncomplicated intoxication
  - Accompanied by a responsible and sober relative/friend
- Offer further help
- No driving

Assessment of alcohol dependence

- CAGE questionnaire (see MICRO-facts)
- More detailed history:
  - Current drinking pattern and for how long?
  - History of alcohol use:
    - Timing of first drink of the day
    - Changes in drink pattern to daily pattern

- Look for evidence of dependence: tolerance over time
- Withdrawal symptoms
- Relief drinking
- Stereotyped pattern
- Compulsion
- Primacy
- Rapid reinstatement after abstinence

MICRO-facts

CAGE questionnaire: Chronic alcohol dependence

1. Do you feel you should **c**ut down on your drinking?
2. Do you feel **a**nnoyed by people criticizing/commenting on your drinking?
3. Do you feel **g**uilty about your drinking?
4. Do you ever need a drink first thing in the morning, an '**e**ye opener' to feel calm or to get rid of a hangover?

>1 positive answer suggests alcohol dependence.
Refer back to GP or local alcohol service (according to local care provision) for a planned detoxification programme in the community.

ALCOHOL WITHDRAWAL

Definition

- Early withdrawal: up to 12 h after the last drink
  - Sweating
  - Fine tremor
  - Anxiety/agitation
  - Nausea and vomiting
- Moderate withdrawal: 12–48 h after last drink
  - More marked autonomic symptoms
  - Alcoholic hallucinosis: auditory hallucinations in clear consciousness
  - Withdrawal seizures

Management

- Seizures: lorazepam up to 4 mg IV
- Education:
  - Explain risks of not drinking
  - Encourage patient to have a drink
- Patient should seek help the following day
- Planned detoxification programme in the community
- No driving
- May need admission to the medical team

Emergency and acute medicine

DELIRIUM TREMENS

Clinical features
- 72 h after the last drink
    - Confusion
    - Aggression/agitation
    - Coarse tremor
    - Autonomic disturbance: profuse sweating, pyrexia
    - Restlessness
    - Fearful
    - Visual hallucinations
    - Illusions

Investigations
- Bloods:
    - FBC (Hb, mean cell volume and platelets)
    - LFTs: ALT, AST, GGT likely to be deranged in chronic alcoholism
    - U&Es: assess for dehydration and potassium levels if acidotic
    - Glucose: hypoglycaemia
    - Clotting screen: may be deranged depending on degree of hepatic impairment
    - Serum phosphate and magnesium
- ECG: arrhythmias
- ABG: metabolic acidosis

Management
- Detain and treat patient under common law
- IV access
- Seizures: lorazepam up to 4 mg IV
- Psychotic symptoms: reducing regimen of chlordiazepoxide
- Thiamine and other vitamins:
    - As IV vitamin B+C (pabrinex)
    - 2 pairs, three times daily
- Treat hypoglycaemia
- Fluid and electrolyte balance
- Admit to care of medical team
- Long term:
    - Specialist referral to psychiatric team
    - Refer to local alcohol services
    - Psychotherapy
    - Rehabilitation

WERNICKE'S ENCEPHALOPATHY

Definition

- Neurological disorder occurring as a result of acute thiamine (vitamin B_1) deficiency
- Characteristically occurs in chronic alcoholism

Clinical features

- Disorientated to time and place
- Nystagmus
- Diplopia
- Ataxia

Management

- IV thiamine and other B vitamins (pabrinex): two pairs of vials 1 and 2, three times daily
- Treat hypoglycaemia: after thiamine administered
- Admit to care of medical team

KORSAKOFF'S PSYCHOSIS

Definition

- Permanent neurological disorder caused by lack of thiamine (vitamin B_1) in the brain

Clinical features

- Antero- or retrograde amnesia
- Confabulation
- Loss of insight
- Apathy
- Ataxia
- Coma

Management

- No specific treatment because thiamine deficiency causes irreversible damage
- Rehabilitation:
  - Replacement of thiamine: oral or IV
  - Improve nutrition
  - Fluids

MICRO-case

A 60-year-old man is brought to the ED by a friend. The friend says he was drunk 3 days ago, fell over and hit his head outside the local pub. He has complained of a worsening headache and vomiting since. He has not had a drink since the fall and since last night has been frightened, sweating, shaking and trying to hit the walls as he thought he could see spiders crawling across them.

On examination, he is disorientated and tachycardic.

He is admitted under the care of the medical team and nursed in a well-lit, quiet room, and given IV fluids and pabrinex.

Key points:

- This man has developed alcohol withdrawal, specifically delirium tremens.
- The complications of alcohol withdrawal are seizures, delirium tremens, Wernicke and Korsakoff psychoses.
- This patient has also suffered a head injury, and this must be treated as well. Due to the worsening headache and vomiting, a CT head would be appropriate as he may have an intracranial bleed.
- It is more appropriate to admit this patient under the medical team and not the psychiatric team, as this is a medical emergency.

19.6 SUBSTANCE ABUSE

Common drugs

- Paracetamol
- Aspirin
- Opioids
- Benzodiazepines
- Tricyclic antidepressants

Clinical features

- A thorough full medical history is important as well as:
  - What was taken and exact amounts? Prescribed or over-the-counter? Own medication or someone else's?
  - How long ago was it taken?
  - Was it taken with another drug or with alcohol?
  - Staggered or all at once?
  - Any vomiting and if so how soon after?
  - Accidental or intentional?
  - Planned or spur of the moment?
  - Final acts?
  - Steps taken to avoid being discovered?

- Witnesses to event?
- Intent to self-harm? Any regrets?
- Persisting suicidal ideation or intent?
- Life stresses/triggers?
- Social support/confidantes?
- Previous history of drug/alcohol/substance abuse?
- Current symptoms if any?
- A collateral history may need to be taken from a relative/friend
- Examination:
  - Some signs are indicative of a particular substance taken, e.g. pinpoint pupils in opioid overdose
  - Formal mental state examination

Investigations

- Full set of observations: monitor for respiratory depression
- Continuous ECG monitoring: particularly following tricyclic antidepressants (prolonged QT interval)
- Bloods:
  - FBC: deranged platelets
  - U&Es: to assess renal function
  - LFTs: may be deranged in chronic alcoholism or paracetamol overdose
  - Clotting screen (specifically PT): deranged clotting in severe paracetamol overdose (marker of prognosis)
  - Serum drug levels: paracetamol, salicylate, etc.
- Urine toxicology screen

Management

- ABCDE including glucose.
- Consult Toxbase® for management advice and guidance.
- Remove drug from system or reverse effect of drug with specific antidote according to guidance.
- Encourage patients to stay until they are risk-free from the drug, even if they feel well. Many drugs taken in overdose may not take effect for a few hours or patients can relapse.
- Risk stratification using the SAD Persons score as highlighted earlier in chapter. Consider referral to the psychiatry team once the patient is medically fit so that a long-term management plan can be established.

19.7 PSYCHOSIS

Definition

- Abnormal condition of the mind with a 'loss of contact with reality'

Emergency and acute medicine

Aetiology

- Organic illness:
  - Neurological: cerebral tumour
  - Endocrine: hypothyroidism
  - Infection: syphilis, HIV
  - Metabolic: hypoglycaemia, hyponatraemia, hypercalcaemia
- Substance abuse:
  - Amphetamines
  - Cocaine
  - Alcohol
- Acute psychosis:
  - Schizophrenia
  - Depression
  - Bipolar disorder
  - Postpartum

MICRO-facts

It is important to exclude organic causes of psychosis before making a diagnosis of a psychiatric disorder.

Clinical features

- Hallucinations: auditory/visual (visual usually organic)
- Delusional beliefs: delusional perception
- Thought disorder: thought withdrawal/insertion/broadcast

Investigations

- Mental state examination
- Bloods:
  - FBC: raised WCC in infection
  - U&Es: low Na; assess renal function
  - LFTs: may be deranged if alcohol or drug related
  - TFTs: low TSH, raised free T3 and T4 (hypothyroidism)
  - Inflammatory markers: raised ESR and CRP in a septic patient
  - Calcium: raised calcium
  - Glucose: low glucose
  - Syphilis serology
  - Consider requesting HIV test
- Urine toxicology screen
- CT/MRI brain and lumbar puncture (LP) if clinically indicated

Management

- Exclude organic cause first
- Urgent psychiatric referral if psychotic symptoms
- Benzodiazepines are the first-line treatment in controlling distressing symptoms: lorazepam 1–2 mg PO/IV/IM
- Admission if loss of insight
- Biological:
  - Antipsychotic medication
  - Electroconvulsive therapy (ECT) if severe/patient at risk
- Psychological therapy

Complications

- Recurrence
- Deliberate self-harm

19.8 DELIRIUM

Definition

- Acute confusional state (usually in the elderly)

Clinical features

- Confusion
- Disorientation
- Clouding of consciousness
- Rapid onset with fluctuating course

Aetiology

- Hypoxia
- Hypoglycaemia
- Systemic infection: respiratory, UTI
- Drug intoxication/withdrawal
- Gross metabolic disturbance
- Vitamin deficiency
- Primary cerebral:
  - Tumours
  - Infection
  - Abscess
  - Haematoma
  - Subarachnoid haemorrhage (SAH)
  - Trauma
- Postictal state
- Myocardial infarction

Investigations

- Mini Mental State Examination (MMSE): interpret according to age and baseline mental state (<9 points/30 is severe cognitive impairment, 10–20 moderate, 21–24 mild and 25 and above is normal)
- Full baseline observations: pulse, NIBP, SpO_2 and respiratory rate
- ABG: metabolic acidosis
- ECG: features of infarct
- CT head: evidence of intracranial bleed, SAH
- Bloods:
  - FBC: raised WCC may indicate infection as cause of delirium
  - U&Es: dehydration and renal impairment
  - Inflammatory markers: raised in sepsis
  - Calcium and phosphate
  - LFTs: liver failure
  - TFTs: uncontrolled hypothyroidism
  - Glucose: hypoglycaemia
- Septic screen:
  - Plain chest radiograph (chest radiograph)
  - Urinalysis: urine dipstick, microscopy, culture and sensitivity
  - Blood cultures
- Cardiac markers: troponin

MICRO-facts

Mini mental state examination

Orientation
- What day, date, month, year, season is it? (5 marks).
- Where are we now? Department, hospital, town, county, country (5 marks).

Registration
- Examiner names three objects e.g. apple, penny, table.
- Patient repeats three objects back (3 marks) and is asked to remember names.

Attention and calculation
- Spell *world* backwards or 100 minus serial sevens (× 5) (5 marks).

Recall
- Repeat three objects from earlier (3 marks).

Language
- Correctly name two identified objects e.g. pencil and watch (2 marks).
- Repeat no ifs, ands or buts (1 mark).

continued...

continued...

- Three-stage command with 1 point for each correct part; take this piece of paper with your right hand, fold it in half and place it on the floor (3 marks).
- Read and obey a written command – close your eyes (1 mark).
- Write a sentence (1 mark).
- Copy a diagram – two intersecting pentagons (1 mark).

Total marks: 30

Management

- Nurse in a well-lit, quiet environment
- Titrated oxygen therapy if hypoxic
- Analgesia
- Ensure adequate hydration – may need IV fluids
- Treat underlying cause
- Stop non-essential medication
- Consider low-dose sedation in distressed/aggressive patients
- Repeat MMSE

Emergency and acute medicine

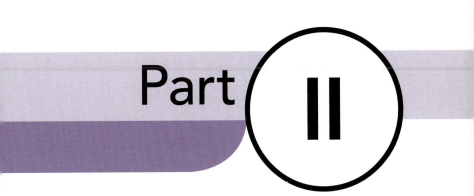

Part II

Self-assessment

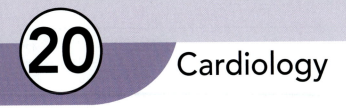

Cardiology

Questions

EMQs

For each of the following questions, please choose the single most likely condition responsible for the presenting conditions. Each option may be used once, more than once or not at all.

Diagnostic options

1. Aortic dissection
2. Costochondritis
3. Musculoskeletal pain
4. NSTEMI
5. Oesophageal spasm
6. Pericarditis
7. Pulmonary embolus
8. Stable angina
9. STEMI
10. Unstable angina

Question 1

i. A 61-year-old man develops central chest pain that is crushing in nature and radiates to his jaw. He is sweating and has vomited once. He is taken to the ED and an ECG shows left bundle branch block (LBBB). This was not evident on an ECG taken 15 min previously.

ii. A 35-year-old woman is referred to the ED with chest pain of gradual onset over the last 24 h. She describes it as stabbing in nature and points to the site of discomfort: a well-localized area on her left anterior chest wall. She notices the pain is relieved on leaning forward. She has suffered with a coryzal illness in the past 2 weeks.

iii. A 50-year-old man develops chest pain after a session at the gym. He attends the ED in an anxious state. On examination he is tachycardic and his sternum is tender. An ECG is normal and troponin is within normal range after 12 h.

SBAs

Question 1

An 80-year-old man is brought to the ED after waking up in the night gasping for breath. He has been sleeping with four pillows recently. On arrival, he is sweating, very pale and very short of breath. On examination, he has an elevated jugular venous pressure (JVP), bibasal crackles on auscultation of his chest and a displaced apex beat. He is treated for acute-on-chronic heart failure. Which of the following is the most appropriate initial management for this patient?

1. Immediate treatment requires non-invasive ventilation (NIV).
2. Keep the patient lying flat.
3. Treat with intravenous loop diuretics, e.g. furosemide.
4. Resuscitate the patient with IV fluids.
5. Treat in the acute setting with beta-blockers to lower BP.

Question 2

A 74-year-old woman has a fall at home and is found by her neighbour. An ambulance is called out to her home and she is taken to the ED. She explains that she felt lightheaded before collapsing. An ECG is performed which shows a heart rate of 38 and is indicative of a third degree heart block. In a patient with bradycardia, which one of the following is correct?

1. Adrenaline is the immediate treatment for a heart rate of <40 bpm.
2. Asymptomatic patients do not require treatment.
3. Complete HB requires urgent treatment only if symptomatic.
4. ECG indicative of a third degree heart block indicates that the patient should be artificially paced.
5. Syncope is an uncommon symptom of bradycardia.

Question 3

A 28-year-old final-year medical student attends the ED in an anxious state complaining of episodes of palpitations lasting for a few minutes over the last few weeks. During this episode they lasted for longer than usual and she felt lightheaded. For this history, which one of the following is most likely?

1. An ECG only needs to be performed if the patient is symptomatic.
2. Atrial fibrillation is the most common cause.
3. Episodes lasting 24 h require cardioversion.
4. ECGs can appear normal.
5. Routine blood tests include cardiac markers.

Question 4

A 60-year-old woman has been experiencing palpitations and mild chest pains for a few months. She has been increasingly hot, sweating and anxious. She attended the ED after feeling lightheaded. An ECG was performed which showed an irregularly irregular rhythm and absent P waves. In patients who present with atrial fibrillation, which one of the following is the most appropriate step?

1. Anticoagulation is only reserved for permanent AF.
2. Electrical cardioversion is required to terminate.
3. First-line treatment is digoxin.
4. Rate control with a calcium channel blocker or beta-blocker may be sufficient to control stable AF.
5. TFTs should always be part of routine blood tests as they are typically abnormal.

Answers

EMQ ANSWERS

Answer 1

i. **(9) STEMI.** The presenting symptoms and ECG pattern indicate an acute ST elevation MI. LBBB is a common finding in older patients and may be chronic; therefore always refer to previous ECGs. This patient should be given symptomatic pain relief, aspirin, put on oxygen and referred to the cardiac catheter lab for emergency PCI. Troponin levels should be taken at 12 h, which would likely show a rise.

ii. **(6) Pericarditis.** This patient has pericarditis. The pain is well localized and sharp in nature, making ischaemic chest pain unlikely. Pain from a pulmonary embolus may be similar in character, but would not be relieved on lying forward. Pericarditis may be associated with a recent viral infection. ECG may demonstrate widespread saddle-shaped (concave) ST elevation if there is concomitant myocarditis, which is common. A clinical diagnosis of pericarditis can be made without ECG changes if there is no myocardial involvement and the history is highly suggestive.

iii. **(3) Musculoskeletal pain.** Due to the age and gender of the patient, all sinister causes of chest pain must be excluded; however, the history of over-exertion, tenderness of the sternum and normal investigation findings are reassuring and the cause is most likely to be of musculoskeletal origin. The tachycardia on examination is likely to be anxiety.

SBA ANSWERS

Answer 1

(3) Treat with intravenous loop diuretics, e.g. furosemide. This patient has signs and symptoms of decompensated heart failure with orthopnoea and paroxysmal nocturnal dyspnea, an elevated JVP and bibasal crepitations.

Fluid overload is a key problem for this patient, and therefore the most important initial management listed would be intravenous diuretic therapy to offload the left ventricle and therefore improve cardiac output. This should also help resolve his pulmonary oedema. IV fluids are not indicated as the patient has fluid overload. Beta-blockers are an evidence-based therapy for chronic stable heart failure, but may make the patient worse in the acute setting, particularly if they have significant pulmonary oedema. They should therefore be avoided. The patient should be kept upright to relieve respiratory symptoms. NIV can be effective in patients to improve pulmonary oedema but this is not immediate treatment.

Answer 2

(4) **ECG indicative of a third-degree heart block indicates that the patient should be artificially paced.** A third-degree heart block is potentially serious and, left unpaced, can lead to haemodynamic instability. A patient may have a heart rate of less than 40 and still be asymptomatic. Although the patient should be treated and not the ECG, the patient may become unwell quickly, and therefore may require early treatment to avoid a sudden deterioration, but consult a senior if in doubt. Atropine is the first-line treatment for unstable bradycardia. Syncope is a fairly common symptom in patients with bradycardia and should always be investigated. Referral to a cardiologist for consideration of a pacemaker would be important for this patient.

Answer 3

(4) **ECGs can appear normal.** Palpitations can be episodic and short lasting; therefore an ECG that is taken between episodes can appear normal. Any patient that presents with palpitations should have an ECG as a minimum investigation, as evidence of a possible cause for the symptom may be seen, e.g. delta wave in Wolff-Parkinson-White syndrome. Not all patients with palpitations require cardioversion; this is for patients with persistent or paroxysmal AF for more than 7 days or unstable arrhythmias where the patient is unwell. Cardiac markers are not part of routine testing and should only be performed if cardiac damage suspected, following MI, etc. This would be extremely uncommon in a young patient. The most common causes in this age group are ectopic beats and sinus tachycardia, although supraventricular tachycardias such as AVNRTs may be seen. AF is commoner in older patients.

Answer 4

(4) **Rate control with a calcium channel blocker or beta-blocker may be sufficient to control stable AF.** Rate control may be sufficient to reverse AF if the patient is stable and usually takes precedence over rhythm control drugs, as these do not work in all cases. Electrical cardioversion should only be reserved for unstable AF and after chemical cardioversion has failed.

TFTs can be abnormal if thyrotoxicosis is the cause for AF; however, this is not the most common cause. Digoxin is not a first-line treatment. Anticoagulation is important to prevent the risk of clot development and complications such as a TIA or a stroke. Paroxysmal AF carries the same risk of stroke as permanent AF, so patients with any history of the arrhythmia should be assessed for anticoagulation with CHADS2-VASc score or similar.

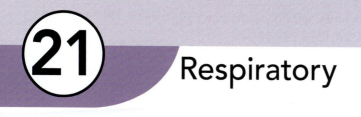

Respiratory

Questions

EMQs

Stem 1 Diagnostic options

1. Acute moderate asthma
2. Acute severe asthma
3. COPD exacerbation
4. Life-threatening asthma
5. Pericarditis
6. Pneumonia
7. Primary spontaneous pneumothorax
8. Pulmonary embolism
9. Secondary spontaneous pneumothorax
10. Tension pneumothorax

Question 1

A 20-year-old man presents to the ED with sudden-onset shortness of breath and right-side chest pain, which is worse on inspiration. On auscultation, breath sounds are decreased on the right when compared to the left. His heart rate is 65 bpm and his blood pressure is 120/70. What is the most likely diagnosis?

Question 2

A 40-year-old woman with known asthma presents to the ED with increased shortness of breath, which is not improved by her reliever (salbutamol). She is mildly distressed, but able to finish her sentences. Her peak expiratory flow (PEF) measurement is 60% of her usual measurement. What is the most likely diagnosis?

Question 3

A 60-year-old woman presents to the ED with sudden-onset shortness of breath and chest pain, which is worse on inspiration. She is currently undergoing chemotherapy treatment for breast cancer. Her pulse is 110 bpm and she has a SpO_2 of 93%. On auscultation, her breath sounds are normal. Her ECG shows sinus tachycardia. You examine her leg and find no signs of

DVT, but on further questioning she reveals that she had a DVT 1 year ago. What is the most likely diagnosis?

Stem 2 Diagnostic options

1. Arterial blood gas	6. ECG
2. Chest X-ray	7. Full blood count
3. CRP	8. Leg vein Doppler
4. CTPA	9. Peak expiratory flow
5. D-dimer	10. Urine antigen

Question 4

A 16-year-old male with known asthma presents with shortness of breath. He is struggling to catch his breath and is unable to complete long sentences. What is the first investigation you would like to do to assess his condition?

Question 5

A 50-year-old male van driver presents with a painful, swollen right leg. He has unilateral pitting oedema and his affected leg measures 4 cm greater than the other. What investigation would you like to do to assess his condition?

Question 6

An 85-year-old woman presents with confusion and shortness of breath. On examination, you hear coarse crepitations and elicit dullness to percussion at the base of her left lung. You suspect she may have pneumonia. What investigation must you do to confirm your diagnosis?

SBAs

Question 1

A 54-year-old woman presents to the ED with pneumonia. She is not confused, but her blood pressure is 85/60 and her respiratory rate is 32. Blood tests show she has a serum urea of 9 mmol/L. What is her CURB65 score?

1. 1 point
2. 2 points
3. 3 points
4. 4 points
5. 5 points

Question 2

A 30-year-old woman presents with sudden onset, increasing shortness of breath with associated pleuritic chest pain. Her heart rate is 110 bpm and her blood pressure is 90/60. She is becoming increasingly distressed. An ABG shows that she is hypoxic. On examination, her trachea is deviated and her right lung shows decreased expansion. What treatment does she need immediately?

1. Analgesia
2. Chest decompression
3. Chest drain
4. Pleural aspirate
5. High-flow oxygen

Question 3

A known asthmatic presents to the ED with shortness of breath. He is unable to finish his sentences, but his chest is clear. The patient's PEF is 50% of normal value. You have given him high-flow oxygen. What is the next treatment you should start?

1. Aminophylline
2. Ipratropium bromide
3. Magnesium sulphate
4. Prednisolone
5. Salbutamol nebulizer

Answers

EMQ ANSWERS

Answer 1

(7) **Primary spontaneous pneumothorax.** Pneumothorax classically presents with sudden onset, pleuritic chest pain and absent breath sounds on auscultation. Pulmonary embolism presents similarly, but without decreased breath sounds and is an unlikely diagnosis in such a young man without significant tachycardia. It is most likely to be a primary spontaneous pneumothorax due to the patient's young age and lack of comorbidities. Secondary pneumothoraces are seen in older patients with chronic lung diseases such as COPD or cancer. Finally, it is unlikely to be tension pneumothorax as his blood pressure and heart rate are stable and normal.

Answer 2

(1) **Acute moderate asthma.** This woman is known to have asthma, which is no longer controlled by her usual medication. Acute moderate asthma is defined as increasing asthma symptoms associated with a reduction in peak expiratory flow (PEF) of 50–75%, but no features of severe asthma.

This woman has a PEF of 60% and is able to finish her sentences. She therefore fits the category of acute moderate asthma.

Answer 3

(8) **Pulmonary embolism (PE).** Sudden-onset shortness of breath associated with inspiratory chest pain can suggests a diagnosis of both PE and pneumothorax. In pneumothorax, you would expect to find areas of absent air entry, which this woman does not have. She has several risk factors for PE, including cancer and previous DVT. She is also very tachycardic, which is the most common finding in PE. She would score 10 on the Wells criteria, making PE the most likely cause, to be ruled out by CTPA.

Answer 4

(9) **Peak expiratory flow.** Peak expiratory flow measurement is the most valuable investigation you can do in any conscious patient suffering from an exacerbation of asthma. It allows you to calculate the percentage of function lost in the episode, which in turn allows you to objectively judge the severity of the episode and to plan treatment. An ABG may be useful in severe or prolonged episodes as it allows analysis of a patient's ability to perform gas exchange. A chest X-ray and a full blood count may be utilized in patients with suspected pneumonia.

Answer 5

(8) **Leg vein Doppler scan.** This is a classical presentation of deep vein thrombosis. The patient's Wells score is 3: pain, pitting oedema and swelling greater than 3 cm compared with the contralateral leg. As such, he is high risk for DVT and the guidelines would recommend proceeding directly to Doppler ultrasound. D-dimer is recommended as the initial test in low to moderate risk of DVT. CTPA may be used to rule out pulmonary embolism, but this man does not display any symptoms of this condition.

Answer 6

(2) **Chest X-ray.** The first investigation for pneumonia is a chest X-ray as it allows you to visualize the area of infective consolidation. A raised white cell count on FBC or a raised CRP will help to confirm the underlying infective process, but cannot localize the infection to the lungs. A urine antigen test may be used to diagnose specific organisms such as *Legionella* spp., but would only be used in rare cases.

SBA ANSWERS

Answer 1

(3) **3 points.** The CURB65 score is made up of five criteria: confusion, raised urea level, high respiratory rate, hypotension and age over 65. This woman

has three of these criteria. She therefore scores 3 points, which gives her a severe score and a 15% risk of death. It is vital to calculate CURB65 scores in all patients with pneumonia, to allow you to risk stratify them and select appropriate treatment.

Answer 2

(2) **Chest decompression.** This patient has a tension pneumothorax. The only way to reduce this quickly, preventing cardiac arrest, is to perform emergency chest compression by inserting a large-bore cannula into the second intercostal space, mid-clavicular line. A chest drain would be inserted following successful decompression.

Answer 3

(5) **Salbutamol nebulizer.** This patient has acute severe asthma, as demonstrated by a PEF of 50% of normal and inability to finish sentences. First-line therapy for acute severe asthma is a short-acting β2-agonist such as salbutamol. The quickest and easiest way to deliver this to the patient is by nebulizer. Steroids such as prednisolone should be considered in all patients with acute asthma, but this is not an immediate treatment. The other treatments listed should be discussed with a senior emergency physician.

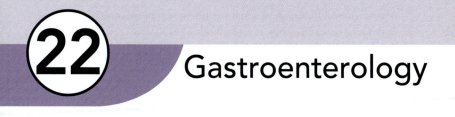

Questions

EMQs

For each of the following questions, please choose the single most likely condition responsible for the presenting conditions. Each option may be used once, more than once or not at all.

Diagnostic options

1. Coagulopathy
2. Drug related
3. Epistaxis
4. Gastritis
5. *H. pylori* infection
6. Mallory-Weiss tear
7. Oesophageal cancer
8. Oesophageal varices
9. Oesophagitis
10. Peptic ulcer

Question 1

i. A 52-year-old man presents to the ED with epigastric pain and an episode of vomiting. During initial assessment in ED he suddenly vomits a large amount of fresh blood and collapses. On examination he has a distended abdomen with prominent veins.

ii. A 38-year-old man presents, anxious after passing black tarry stools. He describes a 6-month history of heartburn and bloating, relieved by antacids.

iii. A 67-year-old woman presents after an episode of vomiting streaked with blood. She has a 3-month history of weight loss, difficulty swallowing food and chest pain.

SBAs

Question 1

A 40-year-old man presents to ED after vomiting blood. As part of the investigation and management of a patient with acute haematemesis, which one of the following is correct?

1. Always give a PPI as part of intial treatment before endoscopy.
2. Arrange urgent endoscopy prior to fluid resuscitation to elicit the cause.
3. Fluid resuscitation should be with 5% dextrose.
4. Assess for signs of chronic liver disease.
5. The risk of re-bleed is increased in younger patients.

Question 2

A 29-year-old woman attends ED after finding bright red blood on the tissue after going to the toilet. In a young patient with an episode of rectal bleeding, which one management plan would be most appropriate?
1. Requires urgent endoscopy to exclude upper GI bleed.
2. Do not perform PR exam if haemorrhoids are suspected.
3. History and examination are sufficient.
4. Perform proctoscopy and PR exam to identify source of bleed.
5. Perform urgent colonoscopy.

Answers

EMQ ANSWERS

Answer 1

i. **(8) Oesophageal varices.** Epigastric pain is typical of an oesophageal cause. This could also be pancreatic, gastritis or of cardiac origin, but with the additional history of massive haematemesis, oesophageal varices are more likely. The swollen abdomen with distended veins indicates chronic liver disease. A Mallory-Weiss tear does not usually present with such a large amount of blood.

ii. **(10) Peptic ulcer.** Black tarry stools indicate an upper GI bleed. The stools are black because the blood is digested as it moves through the GI tract. This is more likely to be a peptic ulcer because of the history of heartburn and bloating, although endoscopy should be performed to confirm this.

iii. **(7) Oesophageal cancer.** In a patient of this age and a history of weight loss and poor swallowing, always be suspicious of malignancy. The chest pain could be retrosternal, cardiac or due to local invasion of anatomically related structures. An endoscopy should always be performed and a CT thorax considered.

SBA ANSWERS

Answer 1

(4) **Assess for signs of chronic liver disease.** Liver disease can often be the underlying cause of acute haematemesis and a careful history and examination is required. It is usually more appropriate to perform endoscopy before giving a PPI. Resuscitation takes priority over endoscopy. Five percent dextrose should not be used for fluid resuscitation as it leaves the intravascular compartment rapidly, and therefore has limited volume-expanding capacity. The risk of re-bleed is increased in older patients (refer to Rockall score in main text).

Answer 2

(4) **Perform proctoscopy and PR exam to identify source of bleed.** Bright red rectal bleeding is unlikely to be upper GI related unless it is an acutely massive bleed. A digital rectal examination may be performed if internal haemorrhoids are suspected. It is not enough to just perform a history and examination for a patient with bleeding; some investigative work must be done. Bloods should be taken and consider urine and stool culture. An urgent colonoscopy should not be performed in patients with acute bleeding because of the risk of causing further bleeds.

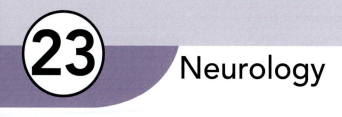

Questions

EMQs

For each of the following questions, please choose the single most likely condition responsible for the presenting conditions. Each option may be used once, more than once or not at all.

Stem 1 Diagnostic options

1. Cluster headache
2. Meningitis
3. Migraine
4. Raised intracranial pressure
5. Stroke
6. Subarachnoid haemorrhage
7. Temporal arteritis
8. Tension headache
9. Transient ischaemic attack (TIA)
10. Trigeminal neuralgia

Question 1

A 30-year-old woman presents to ED with headache. She reports that it came on suddenly, as if she had been hit on the back of the head. She describes it as the worst headache she has ever experienced.

Question 2

A 50-year-old man presents to ED with headache. He has been having multiple episodes of headache over the past few days. The headaches wake him up from sleep and are not relieved by paracetamol. The pain is one sided, centred around his right eye.

Question 3

A 65-year-old women presents to ED with a 4-day history of headache. The pain is worse when she wakes up and is exacerbated by lying down. The pain has become worse today and she has been vomiting.

Stem 2 Diagnostic options

1. Alcohol withdrawal	6. Epileptic seizure
2. Arrhythmic syncope	7. Shock
3. Hyperglycaemia	8. Stroke
4. Hypoglycaemia	9. Transient ischaemic attack
5. Mechanical fall	10. Vasovagal syncope

Question 4

A 20-year-old woman presents to ED following a collapse at work. She is normally fit and well. She experienced a 'flushed' sensation and felt light-headed prior to losing consciousness. Her colleague reports that she collapsed suddenly and recovered within a few seconds.

Question 5

A 60-year-old woman presents to ED following a collapse while walking to the shops. She reports experiencing palpitations and dizziness before blacking out. Her ECG shows runs of non-sustained VT.

Question 6

A 75-year-old woman presents to ED following a fall at home 2 days ago. She reports experiencing leg weakness before she fell and she was unable to use her right arm to steady herself. She reports that this weakness has not entirely improved. On examination she has reduced power and increased tone in her right arm and leg. Her blood glucose is 6 mmol/L.

SBAs

Question 1

A 20-year-old woman is brought to ED in an ambulance and is having a seizure. So far, her seizure has lasted 15 min. What treatment should you give her immediately?

1. Diazepam PR
2. Lorazepam IV
3. Pabrinex IV
4. Phenobarbital IV
5. Phenytoin IV

Question 2

A 30-year-old man presents to ED with headache, neck stiffness and photophobia. The results of a lumbar puncture show xanthacromia and red blood cells. What is the most likely diagnosis?

1. Bacterial meningitis
2. Subarachnoid haemorrhage
3. Subdural haemorrhage
4. TB meningitis
5. Viral meningitis

Question 3

A 60-year-old woman taking warfarin for atrial fibrillation falls and bangs her head. She sustained no other injuries, but her speech has now become slurred. You perform a CT scan. What are you expecting to see?
1. Intracranial bleeding
2. Cerebral atrophy
3. Cerebral mass
4. Ischaemic changes
5. Normal scan

Answers

EMQ ANSWERS

Answer 1

(6) **Subarachnoid haemorrhage.** Subarachnoid haemorrhage often presents as a feeling of being hit on the back of the head and patients classically report it as the worst headache they have ever had.

Answer 2

(1) **Cluster headache.** Cluster headaches typically affect men and are often experienced in bouts or 'clusters' of headaches. The pain classically centres around one eye and can be extremely severe and unresponsive to normal pain medication.

Answer 3

(4) **Raised intracranial pressure.** Raised intracranial pressure often presents insidiously over a few days. Any increase to the pressure, such as leaning over, lying down or coughing, exacerbates the pain. At high pressures, vomiting is common and may be intractable.

Answer 4

(10) **Vasovagal syncope.** In a history of falls it is most useful to take into account what is observed by others. This woman's colleagues describe that she collapsed and was unconscious for only a few seconds. The short, uncomplicated duration

makes a seizure unlikely and a woman of this age is extremely unlikely to have had a stroke or a TIA. It is most likely that this is a case of syncope. In absence of cardiac disease, it is unlikely to be arrhythmic syncope and vasovagal syncope is often preceeded by a flushing sensation and light-headedness.

Answer 5

(2) **Arrhythmic syncope.** Unfortunately, there is no eyewitness account of this woman's fall, but her description of palpitations and dizziness preceeding her collapse is highly suggestive of cardiac arrhythmia leading to haemodynamic compromise and syncope. Non-sustained VT commonly presents with syncope, and her ECG confirms the presence of this arrhythmia.

Answer 6

(8) **Stroke.** This woman's conscious loss of function preceeding her collapse could have been caused by either a TIA, stroke or hypoglycaemia, but the episode occurred 2 days ago and she has residual weakness. This rules out TIA, which by definition resolves within 24 h, and hypoglycaemia, which does not result in unresolved weakness.

SBA ANSWERS

Answer 1

(1) **Diazepam PR.** This woman has already been fitting for 15 min. You therefore need to attempt to stop the seizure as soon as possible. Rectal diazepam may be given immediately, while you are gaining IV access to allow use of other drugs.

Answer 2

(2) **Subarachnoid haemorrhage.** Xanthochromia (yellow colour) is caused by the presence of blood in the CSF and is the typical finding in subarachnoid haemorrhage. Red blood cells confirm that there is blood in the CSF. Subdural haemorrhage would not result in blood in the CSF, while the presence of TB or bacterial meningitis would result in a turbid appearance. The CSF is often clear in viral meningitis.

Answer 3

(1) **Intracranial bleeding.** This woman has a high risk of bleeding due to taking warfarin. Loss of function following a blow to the head is therefore likely to be caused by haemorrhage. This would show up as blood on a CT scan. Atrial fibrillation increases the risk of emboli to the brain, which might result in ischaemic changes; however, this patient is warfarinized and therefore less likely to present this way.

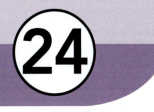

Endocrinology and electrolyte abnormalities

Questions

EMQs

For each of the questions, select the most likely option from the list below. Answers can be used once, more than once or not at all.

Diagnostic options

1. Diabetic ketoacidosis (DKA)
2. Hypercalcaemia
3. Hyperosmolar hyperglycaemic state (HHS)
4. Hypernatraemia
5. Hypoglycaemia
6. Hypermagnasaemia
7. Metabolic acidosis
8. Metabolic alkalosis
9. Rhabdomyolysis
10. Transient ischaemic attack (TIA)

Question 1

i. You are the FY2 in the ED. You are asked to see a 15-year-old male with Down syndrome who has become increasingly aggressive over the past few hours. His mother tells you that he is usually very calm but that he has been behaving strangely this morning. He is sweaty and anxious and is complaining that his vision is blurry. His mother tells you that he has type I diabetes. He has been to the ED with DKA before, but his mother insists that she gave him his regular insulin this morning. His blood glucose is 2.4 mmol/L. The patient then tells you that he wasn't feeling well this morning, so did not eat his breakfast.

ii. A 75-year-old woman is brought to the ED after being found on the floor by her daughter. The patient is confused and cold. No one is aware how long she was on the floor. She is admitted to the ward, a full confusion screen is performed and blood tests show a potassium level of 7.1 mmol/L.

iii. During your medical night shifts, you are called to see a 70-year-old woman who has become increasingly confused in the middle of the night and is complaining of ongoing abdominal pain. She was admitted with a pathological fracture of her humeral head. She has no other significant medical history of note other than hypertension and previous right mastectomy.

SBAs

Question 1

What are the three most important lines of intervention when treating a case of DKA?
1. Fluids, insulin and sodium
2. Fluids, insulin and potassium
3. Fluids, glucose and potassium
4. Insulin, potassium and bicarbonate
5. Insulin, potassium and enoxaparin

Question 2

In hypoglycaemia, why is it important to continue insulin treatment in type I diabetics?
1. To decrease their serum glucose
2. To increase their serum glucose
3. To avoid precipitation of DKA
4. To maintain potassium levels
5. To prevent development of HHS

Question 3

Why should caution be taken in hypokalaemic patients who are on digoxin?
1. Can precipitate a cerebral event
2. Can lead to nausea and vomiting
3. May result in hyperglycaemia
4. Causes hyperviscosity
5. Can cause blindness

Question 4

Addison's disease can cause the following:
1. Weight gain, hypernatraemia and hypokalaemia
2. Weight loss, hypernatraemia and hypercalcaemia
3. Thirst, hyponatraemia and hyperkalaemia
4. Weight loss, hyponatraemia and hyperkalaemia
5. Vision change, hyponatraemia and hyperkalaemia

Question 5

In the management of hyponatraemia, it is essential to:
1. Correct the deficiency rapidly.
2. Always ensure it is treated.
3. Avoid rapid correction of the deficiency.
4. Administer calcium resonium.
5. Ensure that a cardiac monitor is attached.

Question 6

Hypercalcaemia can occur when malignancies metastasize to the bone. This is more common in:
1. Testicular cancer
2. Oesophageal cancer
3. Breast cancer
4. Liver cancer
5. Pancreatic cancer

Answers

EMQ ANSWERS

Answer 1

i. **(5) Hypoglycaemia.** In those treated with insulin, it is vital that meals are regular and of an adequate size. If not, insulin treatment results in hypoglycaemia. Symptoms like aggression and visual disturbance occur at extremely low blood glucose levels. Poor glycaemic control is very common in young people who have recently been diagnosed with diabetes. It is paramount that both the individual and their parents/carers understand the condition and its management. The ED can be very busy, and it can be difficult to spend time with a family discussing such things, but even a small amount of discussion can be beneficial and may prevent future admissions. Type I diabetes is commonly associated with Down syndrome.

ii. **(9) Rhabdomyolysis.** Given the history, the most likely cause is rhabdomyolysis, which is extensive muscle damage which results in the release of myoglobin; this is toxic to renal tubular cells which results in acute renal failure due to the release of potassium into the circulation. This woman has been on the floor for an unknown period of time, and as a result would have suffered from muscle damage. Her potassium level will need treating immediately, as hyperkalaemia can be fatal.

iii. **(2) Hypercalcaemia.** This patient was admitted having had a pathological fracture. Metastatic bone disease increases the risk of developing pathological fractures. The most common malignancies that can cause bony metastases are breast, bronchus, thyroid, prostate and kidney. Note the previous mastectomy. Bony metastases result in hypercalcaemia which can cause confusion and abdominal pain.

SBA ANSWERS

Answer 1

(2) **Fluids, insulin and potassium.** Hyperglycaemia causes an osmotic diuresis and acidosis can lead to vomiting. Both of these factors contribute to fluid depletion. Fluids must be replaced using normal saline (NaCl 0.9%). Insulin acts to restore normal serum glucose. If the treatment is adequate, serum glucose should decrease by 5 mmol/L/h. Insulin therapy leads to the general uptake of potassium ions by cells in the body, leading to fall in serum potassium levels. For this reason, potassium therapy, in the form of KCl, must be commenced as soon as insulin therapy is started.

Answer 2

(3) **To avoid precipitation of DKA.** People with type I diabetes have no endogenous production of insulin, unlike the normal population and those with type II diabetes, who retain some function. After restoring their serum glucose to a normal level, they require insulin treatment to prevent refractory hyperglycaemia and thus DKA. It may, however, be the case that their dose needs to be lowered. Discuss this with a diabetes specialist.

Answer 3

(2) **Can cause nausea and vomiting.** Hypokalaemia can predispose a patient taking digoxin to developing digoxin toxicity. Digoxin competes with K^+ ions for the same binding site. Features of digoxin toxicity include anorexia, nausea, vomiting, blurred vision, xanthopsia and reverse tick shape ECG changes in ST segment.

Answer 4

(4) **Weight loss, hyponatraemia and hyperkalaemia.** Addison's disease is a result of the autoimmune destruction of the adrenal cortex. The adrenal cortex is responsible for making glucocorticoids (cortisol), androgens and mineralocorticoids (aldosterone). Cortisol leads to increased fat and glycogen deposition, protein catabolism. Aldosterone causes increased renal potassium loss and sodium retention. In the absence of these hormones, the opposite occurs – hence the reduced fat deposition, potassium retention and sodium loss.

Answer 5

(3) **Avoid rapid correction of the deficiency.** Rapid correction of hyponatraemia can lead to central pontine myelinolysis. This is a neurological condition caused by local areas of demyelination resulting in paralysis, respiratory arrest and seizures. Mild hyponatraemia does not always need correction.

Answer 6

(3) **Breast cancer.** Breast, bronchus, thyroid, prostate and renal malignancies most commonly metastasize to bone. Bony metastases result in hypercalcaemia as they cause resorption of the bone, releasing calcium.

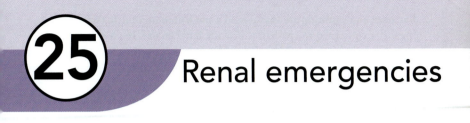

Renal emergencies

Questions

EMQs

For each of the following questions, please choose the single most likely condition responsible for the presenting conditions. Each option may be used once, more than once or not at all.

Diagnostic options

1. Acute pyelonephritis
2. Appendicitis
3. Benign prostatic hypertrophy
4. Ectopic pregnancy
5. Lower lobe pneumonia
6. Musculoskeletal back pain
7. Renal stones
8. Ruptured AAA
9. Testicular torsion
10. UTI

Question 1

i. A 32-year-old woman develops pain in her right loin that radiates to the right iliac fossa and suprapubic region. She has had four episodes of vomiting over the last 24 h and has dysuria, rigors and fever.

ii. A 19-year-old female visits her GP complaining of lower abdominal pain and dysuria for the past 2 days. She is also concerned she might be pregnant after having unprotected sex but cannot remember the date of her last menstrual period. A urine dipstick test is positive for blood, leucocytes and nitrites.

iii. A 48-year-old man presents to the ED with sudden onset of severe pain that comes in waves in his left loin that radiates to the testes. On examination, he is tender in his left loin.

SBAs

Question 1

A 71-year-old man is sent to the ED after routine blood tests at his GP surgery show high elevation of his creatinine levels. The patient has recently had diarrhoea and vomiting and has passed a small amount of urine over 24 h. The GP is concerned the patient is in acute renal failure. In an elderly male with acute renal failure, which of the following is correct?

1. A typical ECG will show features of hypokalaemia.
2. Metabolic acidosis is a potential complication.
3. On clinical examination, it is not appropriate to perform a rectal examination.
4. Fluid resuscitation is always indicated in renal failure.
5. Urine dipstick testing is not helpful in this case.

Question 2

A 21-year-old woman attends the ED with lower back pain, pain on passing urine and feels feverish. A test is done which confirms a UTI. In a young woman with an uncomplicated lower UTI, which one of the following is most likely?

1. A 3- to 5-day course of trimethoprim is an effective treatment.
2. A typical urine dipstick will show positive blood but no nitrites.
3. Chlamydial infection is likely in this patient.
4. Investigation for anatomical abnormalities is always indicated.
5. The most common organism is *Staphylococcus saprophyticus.*

Question 3

A 54-year-old man presents after being unable to pass urine for 24 h. Two days previously, he had a CT angiogram with contrast under the vascular team to investigate his intermittent claudication. A diagnosis of acute renal failure due to contrast-induced nephropathy is made. As part of the investigation and management of acute renal failure, which one of the following is most appropriate?

1. KUB X-ray is an appropriate investigation for assessing and excluding obstruction.
2. Skin turgor is a reliable clinical sign to guide management of fluid therapy.
3. Sodium bicarbonate should always be given.
4. Long-term dialysis is likely to be needed.
5. Urinary catheterization may be indicated to monitor response to treatment.

Question 4

The same patient receives IV fluids but his poor renal function persists, and a decision is made to start haemodialysis. Which of the following are indications for haemodialysis in acute renal failure?

1. Low systolic blood pressure despite fluids
2. Narrow QRS complexes on ECG and a raised potassium

3. Metabolic acidosis with pH 7.0
4. Patients with diabetes mellitus
5. Sepsis

Answers

EMQ ANSWERS

Answer 1

i. **(1) Acute pyelonephritis.** The dysuria, fever and rigors suggest a UTI. This patient should be admitted and have her urine tested for urinalysis, microscopy and culture. She should also have a CT-KUB to look for stones and assess renal function.

ii. **(10) UTI.** The history of lower abdominal pain and dysuria and the results of the dipstick suggest a lower UTI. A pregnancy test should be performed and it would be essential to consider ectopic pregnancy as a differential diagnosis.

iii. **(7) Renal stone.** The sudden onset of this severe pain is most likely to be the result of a stone along the urinary tract. It is, however, important to include testicular torsion in the differential diagnosis as well as infection with obstruction; therefore this patient should have urine testing and CT-KUB.

SBA ANSWERS

Answer 1

(2) **Metabolic acidosis is a potential complication.** Metabolic acidosis is a complication in patients with acute renal failure, and it is important to identify this as it impairs cardiac contractility and oxygen delivery to tissues. If this cannot be corrected, then the patient may require haemodialysis/filtration. Hyperkalaemia is an important complication of acute renal failure. The patient may be fluid overloaded or obstructed; therefore first assess ABC and hydration status and consider a catheter. It may well be appropriate to give IV fluids after this. This is an elderly patient and it is important to exclude obstruction as a cause of his renal failure; therefore examine for masses per rectum to look for an enlarged prostate.

Answer 2

(1) **A 3- to 5-day course of trimethoprim is an effective treatment.** Trimethoprim is effective providing she does not have more systemic symptoms and pregnancy is excluded due to the teratogenicity of the drug. If upper UTI

is suspected, the patient may need to be admitted and should be prescribed cefuroxime. The most common organism in the community is *Escherichia coli*. Chlamydia infection is more likely to present with some vaginal discharge as well as some symptoms of a UTI, but it is often asymptomatic; therefore the patient should be offered screening if she is sexually active. If there are no complications or risk factors and this is her first UTI, then it is not necessary to refer this patient for further investigation. Anatomical abnormalities are also more common in males.

Answer 3

(5) **Urinary catheterization may be indicated to monitor response to treatment.** It is important to measure urine output in management of acute renal failure. If appropriately managed, acute renal failure can be reversible and usually improves over weeks to resume normal baseline renal function. Not all patients have severe enough acidosis to require sodium bicarbonate. Bicarbonate therapy is used only in selective cases and should be administered under specialist care as the patient can be sent into severe hypokalaemia. Skin turgor is a very crude method to assess dehydration and a poor guide to fluid and blood volume. Ultrasound scanning is sensitive for assessing obstruction.

Answer 4

(3) **Metabolic acidosis with pH 7.0.** Dialysis can correct severe metabolic acidosis. It is indicated when pH <7.2. The ECG changes indicative of a severe hyperkalaemia are tented T waves, absent P waves and broad QRS complexes, and are an indication for dialysis if refractory to medical therapy. Sepsis is a cause for acute kidney injury but not an indication for dialysis. A low systolic BP should not be treated with haemodialysis. Fluid bolus would be appropriate, then senior review if unchanged. Diabetes mellitus can increase the risk of developing chronic renal failure with acute exacerbations but is not an indication for dialysis.

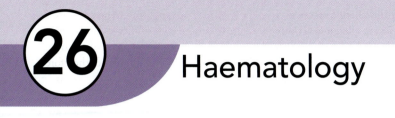

26 Haematology

Questions

SBAs

Question 1

A 56-year-old woman with rheumatoid arthritis treated with methotrexate presents with tiredness. A full blood count shows macrocytic anaemia. What is the most likely cause?

1. Anaemia of chronic disease
2. B_{12} deficiency
3. Folate deficiency
4. Iron deficiency anaemia
5. Haemolytic anaemia

Question 2

A patient with known haemophilia A presents with an open fracture. The haematologist suggests you order blood products for administration. What do you need to request?

1. Cryoprecipitate
2. Factor VIII concentrate
3. Factor IX concentrate
4. Fresh frozen plasma
5. Packed red cells

Question 3

A patient undergoing a blood transfusion spikes a fever of 38° within the first few minutes of receiving the transfusion. You stop the giving set, check all of the details and find that there is no mistake in the blood being delivered. The patient is otherwise well. What is the most likely cause of the patient's pyrexia?

1. ABO incompatability
2. Anaphylaxis
3. Febrile, non-haemolytic transfusion reaction

4. Mild allergic reaction
5. Severe allergic reaction

Answers

SBA ANSWERS

Answer 1

(3) **Folate deficiency.** Anaemia is common in a patient with a chronic disease such as rheumatoid arthritis; however, 'anaemia of chronic disease' typically retains normocytic cells. Macrocytic anaemia may be caused by B_{12} and folate deficiency. In this case, methotrexate, an antifolate drug, has caused folate deficiency.

Answer 2

(2) **Factor VIII concentrate.** Haemophilia A is a congenital deficiency of factor VIII; therefore this is the blood product of choice. Other blood products may be required if there is severe blood loss from the fracture.

Answer 3

(3) **Febrile, non-haemolytic transfusion reaction.** In any patient with fever, a blood transfusion should be stopped immediately and the patient and the blood products fully examined. In this case, the only symptom is fever and there is nothing wrong with the blood, therefore it can be assumed that this is a febrile, non-haemolytic transfusion reaction. The blood transfusion may therefore be continued at a slower rate. In allergic reaction, urticaria, abdominal pain and bronchospasm may be seen. In anaphylaxis, the patient would show signs of airway compromise. An ABO incompatibility reaction is seen in patients given the incorrect blood products. See Chapter 9 for detailed management of these conditions.

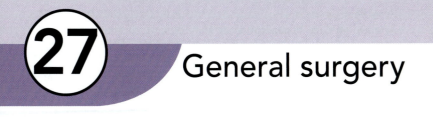

General surgery

Questions

EMQs

For each of the questions, select the most likely option from the list below. Answers can be used once, more than once or not at all.

Diagnostic options

1. Abdominal aortic aneurysm
2. Acute cholecystitis
3. Appendicitis
4. Ascending cholangitis
5. Ectopic pregnancy
6. Large bowel obstruction
7. Pyelonephritis
8. Renal colic
9. Small bowel obstruction
10. Testicular torsion

Question 1

i. A 25-year-old female presents with sudden-onset right iliac fossa pain. She is hypotensive and tachycardic. She has no other medical history other than asthma.

ii. A 38-year-old male presents to the ED with intermittent sharp pain in his right loin. He is finding it impossible to get comfortable, and his urine dipstick has ++ blood. He has no allergies and takes allopurinol.

iii. A 75-year-old woman who is admitted on the orthopaedic ward 5 days after a right hip hemiarthroplasty has not opened her bowels for 7 days. She denies passing flatus and feels bloated and nauseous. She has angina, COPD and previously had an open appendicectomy.

Diagnostic options

For each of the questions, select the most likely option from the list below. Answers can be used once, more than once or not at all.

1. Acute cholecystitis
2. Acute urinary retention
3. Ascending cholangitis
4. Ectopic pregnancy
5. Large bowel obstruction
6. Pyelonephritis

7. Renal colic
8. Retained products of conception
9. Small bowel obstruction
10. Testicular torsion

Question 2

i. A 30-year-old female presents with left flank pain. The pain is constant and achy. She has felt nauseated and reports some fever, urinary frequency and dysuria.

ii. A 53-year-old male attends the ED with worsening right upper quadrant abdominal pain. He is febrile and nauseated. On examination he catches his breath when the painful area is palpated.

iii. A 35-year-old female is 1 day post-partum. She had a forceps delivery of a live healthy male for which she required an epidural. Her urine output has only been 40 mL in the last 24 h. She is complaining of lower abdominal pain.

SBAs

Question 1

A 60-year-old male presents with severe left loin pain which has been worsening over the last few hours. He is feeling nauseated and feverish. He has had similar pain in the past. Which one of the following would not normally be part of the management plan?

1. CT KUB
2. IV antibiotics
3. IV fluids
4. IV steroids
5. Renal tract ultrasound scan

Question 2

A 28-year-old woman is currently 15 weeks pregnant in her third pregnancy. She has had several episodes of intermittent right upper quadrant abdominal pain that radiates into her back. She has a BMI of 38, but is otherwise fit and well. What is the most likely diagnosis?

1. Acute cholecystitis
2. Appendicitis
3. Ascending cholangitis
4. Biliary colic
5. Peptic ulcer disease

Question 3

Which one of the following clinical features is not associated with an ischaemic limb?

1. Loss of hair
2. Muscle wasting

3. Pallor
4. Warmth
5. Reduced sensation

Question 4

A 23-year-old male presents with a tender, warm testicular mass. He has had some mild dysuria but is otherwise systemically well. What is the most likely diagnosis?
1. Hydrocoele
2. Epididymo-orchitis
3. Epididymal cyst
4. Testicular tumour
5. Varicocele

Answers

EMQ ANSWERS

Answer 1

i. **(5) Ectopic pregnancy.** It is always important to perform a pregnancy test in females of childbearing age who present with abdominal pain. If the pregnancy test is negative, appendicitis would be the most likely cause for the pain after an ectopic pregnancy. It is important to remember that pregnant women can still have appendicitis!

ii. **(8) Renal colic.** This patient is a male with gout, which puts him at a higher risk of developing renal calculi. Patients with renal calculi are often in agony and require urgent analgesia. Haematuria often occurs in renal calculi as the renal tract epithelium is damaged by the passing calculi.

iii. **(6) Large bowel obstruction.** This woman has features of lower bowel obstruction in the gastrointestinal tract. If she had presented with vomiting this would have made small bowel obstruction more likely, although vomiting eventually does occur in large bowel obstruction too. She has had previous abdominal surgery which may have resulted in adhesions, which are a risk factor for bowel obstruction. A rectal examination and AXR should be organized.

Answer 2

i. **(6) Pyelonephritis.** This patient has features of an upper urinary tract infection. She is feeling systemically unwell and will need intravenous antibiotics and fluids. She will also need a renal ultrasound scan.

ii. **(1) Acute cholecystitis.** This patient appears to have a positive Murphy sign on examination of the abdomen, which indicates likely acute cholecystitis given his clinical picture. He will need intravenous fluids and antibiotics as well as a surgical review to decide further management.

iii. **(2) Acute urinary retention.** Epidurals are often used for pain relief in labour. This woman has lower abdominal tenderness, and a distended bladder may be palpated. Acute urinary retention can be very uncomfortable and urinary catheterization will usually treat this acute episode. Retained products would be highly unlikely in the case of a forceps vaginal delivery requiring an epidural, as this would have been checked during delivery.

SBA ANSWERS

Answer 1

(4) **IV steroids.** The differential diagnoses include renal calculi, pyelonephritis and abdominal aortic aneurysm. IV fluids would be needed for all these cases and IV antibiotics would be needed for pyelonephritis. Both renal tract ultrasound and CT KUB would be of diagnostic value, but IV steroids have no role in the management of either of these diagnoses.

Answer 2

(4) **Biliary colic.** Biliary colic is the most likely cause in this case and in women who are of a fertile age and overweight. Peptic ulcer disease can also present in a similar manner, but there is not enough information in the case to indicate this.

Answer 3

(4) **Warmth.** Muscle wasting and reduced hair are signs of chronic vascular insufficiency. Reduced sensation and pallor can be present with an acute ischaemic limb as can coolness of the limb, as opposed to warmth.

Answer 4

(2) **Epididymo-orchitis.** It is possible that this patient has an STI, which could account for the epididymo-orchitis, which results in a tender, swollen testicle. Dysuria and urethral discharge may also be present. Chlamydia is a common cause. It is important to rule out testicular torsion as urgent intervention is required for this.

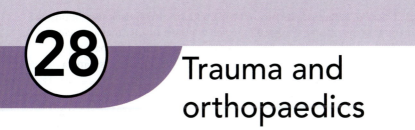

28 Trauma and orthopaedics

Questions

EMQs

For each of the following questions, please choose the single most likely condition responsible for the presenting conditions. Each option may be used once, more than once or not at all.

Diagnostic options

1. Acute gout
2. Dislocation of the patella
3. Meniscal tear
4. Osteoarthritis of the knee
5. Osteomyelitis

6. Pseudogout
7. Reactive arthritis
8. Referred pain
9. Ruptured ACL
10. Septic arthritis

Question 1

i. A 60-year-old man attends the ED after he woke up in the night with severe pain in his right big toe. The toe is red, shiny and extremely tender such that he will not allow anyone to examine it.

ii. A 23-year-old man presents with severe pain in his left knee that came on suddenly while playing rugby. During a tackle, he heard a 'popping' sound and his knee immediately swelled up. He feels his knee 'gives way' while trying to weight bear.

iii. A 42-year-old woman presents with pain in the left knee while skiing. On examination there is an effusion and decreased range of movement and she cannot fully extend the leg. A plain X-ray of the left knee is normal.

SBAs

Question 1

A 34-year-old man presents to the ED 1 day after falling down a flight of stairs at work. He hit his head and blacked out for a few minutes. He went home to rest but has had two episodes of vomiting and a worsening headache.

A CT head is requested. Of the following options, which one is not part of the criteria for requesting a CT head?

1. Two episodes of vomiting
2. GCS <15 when assessed in the ED 2 h after the injury
3. Headache within 24 h of injury
4. Seizure related to head injury
5. Amnesia lasting 1 h after injury

Question 2

A 65-year-old woman is gardening when she trips over her cat and falls onto her hand. Her neighbour takes her to the ED where she is assessed and treated for a fracture. Of the following options, which one is correct about this patient?

1. An X-ray will not always identify the fracture.
2. Neurovascular state only needs to be examined if surgery is considered.
3. This patient has had a Colles fracture.
4. The patient should not move her hand after the fracture for a few weeks, as this will delay healing.
5. The type of fracture can always be determined from the mechanism of injury.

Question 3

A 23-year-old man presents with multiple stab wounds, some of which are on his chest. During initial assessment he develops acute severe dyspnoea and quickly becomes very unwell. A tension pneumothorax is suspected. In a patient with a suspected tension pneumothorax, which one of the following is correct?

1. Request an urgent portable chest X-ray.
2. A trachea deviated to the right-hand side typically suggests a massive right-side tension pneumothorax.
3. The patient becomes tachycardic and hypertensive very quickly.
4. An ABG is normal.
5. Perform urgent chest decompression without a chest radiograph.

Question 4

A 45-year-old man presents with lower back pain after trying to lift a heavy box in his attic. He also has bilateral leg pain and numbness. In patients with lower back pain, which one of the following does not warrant an urgent MRI of the spine?

1. Urinary or bowel disturbance
2. Mechanical back pain
3. Concurrent fever
4. Perineal numbness
5. Bilateral leg pain

Question 5

A 26-year-old woman is involved in a road traffic accident and sustains a femoral and pelvic fracture. When she arrives in hospital, her heart rate is 110 bpm and her blood pressure is 98/56 mmHg and she is on 15 L/min of oxygen via a non-rebreathe mask. Of the following options, which one is correct regarding the initial management?

1. Prescribe pain relief only when the patient feels her pain is severe enough.
2. Give a fluid bolus of 250 mL of 5% dextrose.
3. It is not necessary to obtain a cross-match for blood initially.
4. Early referral to orthopaedics to prepare for theatre following resuscitation.
5. Ordering plain radiographs to establish extent of fracture is the first priority.

Answers

EMQ ANSWERS

Answer 1

i. **(1) Acute gout.** The great toe is a common site for acute gout. Pain is typically severe and on examination, exquisitely tender. A joint aspirate should be performed and on microscopy, typically shows negatively birefringent crystals.

ii. **(9) Ruptured ACL.** This is a classic presentation of a ruptured anterior cruciate ligament. The cause and symptoms are very similar to a meniscal tear; however, the history of immediate swelling following injury and instability of the knee is more typical of ACL rupture.

iii. **(3) Meniscal tear.** Twisting injury is a common mechanism of injury in meniscal tear. The patient may commonly describe locking and an inability to fully extend the knee. An effusion may not develop initially, and therefore may not be evident on early examination.

SBA ANSWERS

Answer 1

(3) **Headache within 24 h of injury.** A headache within the first 24 h alone is not enough of a clinical indication for a CT head without other features. Most head injuries, no matter how minor, will cause some discomfort to the patient initially, and this therefore is not always a good clinical indication. The other options listed indicate more severe consequences of head injury and should be further investigated.

Answer 2

(1) **An X-ray will not always identify the fracture.** Not all fractures (scaphoid in this case) can be identified initially on X-ray; therefore it is important to bring the patient back to fracture clinic for a repeat radiograph. The type of fracture cannot always be identified from the type of injury, although some fractures are more common than others due to the mechanism. Neurovascular state should always be assessed for every fracture as there is always a risk to the distal limb. Early mobilization of the affected limb is important.

Answer 3

(5) **Perform urgent chest decompression without a chest radiograph.** A tension pneumothorax is a life-threatening emergency and requires immediate chest decompression. Do not delay this by ordering a chest radiograph to confirm your clinical findings. An ABG typically shows type 1 respiratory failure with hypoxia, but again, this should not be performed before decompression is attempted. In a large tension pneumothorax, the trachea deviates away from the affected side as the mediastinum is pushed away from the affected lung, but do not rely on this sign alone. The patient often goes into cardiogenic shock and will become hypotensive quickly.

Answer 4

(2) **Mechanical back pain.** Mechanical back pain is less sinister than non-mechanical and does not generally require an urgent MRI. The other options suggest a more threatening cause to the spine and an MRI may be requested with a view to surgery. Neurological features such as bilateral leg pain, urinary or bowel symptoms and numbness require an urgent scan because the consequence of delayed management is permanent neurological damage.

Answer 5

(4) **Early referral to orthopaedics to prepare for theatre following resuscitation.** Resuscitation for early hypovolaemic shock is the priority in this case. It is important to alert the orthopaedic team at an early stage as this patient will require fixation of her fractures and it is important to prepare for theatre. This includes taking the appropriate bloods including a cross-match for at least 4 units of blood. Strong regular analgesia should be prescribed as the patient will undoubtedly be in severe pain, but this also reduces heart and respiratory rate and increases the risk of developing a chest infection due to ineffective breathing as a result of uncontrolled pain. In younger patients, larger fluid boluses can be administered safely without fluid overload. Five percent dextrose is not an ideal resuscitative fluid as it leaves the intravascular space too quickly to have a volume-expanding effect.

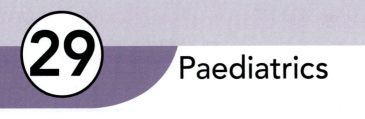

Paediatrics

Questions

EMQs

For each of the questions, select the most likely option from the list of diagnostic options. Answers can be used once, more than once or not at all.

Diagnostic options

1. Appendicitis
2. Bronchiectasis
3. Gastroenteritis
4. Intussusception
5. Lobar pneumonia
6. Migraine
7. Meningococcal meningitis with septicaemia
8. Menstruation
9. Pneumothorax
10. Testicular torsion

Question 1

i. A 7-year-old girl presents to the ED with a 3-day history of fever, lethargy and a productive cough. She has recently returned from a family holiday abroad. She has been off her food and complaining of generalised muscle aches and neck stiffness. On examination, she is tachypnoeic, well hydrated but febrile. A full systemic examination is performed which is essentially normal other than reduced air entry at the left upper lobe.

ii. A 13-year-old girl is brought by her father to the ED with lower abdominal cramps. She has no urinary symptoms and her bowels are normal, however, she has noticed some blood in her underwear. On examination she is normotensive, her abdomen is soft but she is anxious. A urine dip performed contains large amounts of blood.

iii. A 5-year-old boy is rushed to the ED with a 2-day history of lethargy, poor oral intake and poor urinary output. On examination he is drowsy and dislikes the bright ED room. A small area of rash is present on his right upper arm.

Diagnostic options

1. Appendicitis
2. Bronchiolitis
3. Cardiac failure
4. Foreign body
5. Lobar pneumonia
6. Intussusception
7. Meningococcal meningitis
8. Otitis media
9. Tonsillitis
10. Urinary tract infection

Question 2

i. A 2-year-old girl attends with her mother. This morning, she had been playing with her 5-year-old sister, but has since developed a worsening dry cough all day that has not improved. She has been eating and drinking well and is afebrile. On examination there is reduced air entry at the right lung base.

ii. An 8-month-old boy attends the ED with his parents. He has recently had symptoms of a cold. He has become increasingly breathless over the past 2 days with a dry cough, poor oral intake and wheezing.

iii. A 10-year-old female presents with sharp right lower abdominal pain and is feeling nauseated. The pain was initially present around her umbilicus, but has now moved. She is unable to cough and is finding it hard to move.

Diagnostic options

1. Asthma
2. Bronchiolitis
3. Croup
4. Cystic fibrosis
5. Diphtheria
6. Epiglottitis
7. Foreign body inhalation
8. Lobar pneumonia
9. Quinsy
10. Tonsillitis

Question 3

i. A 6-year-old boy presents with a severe sore throat and fever. On examination there is soft stridor. He is unable to drink or swallow his saliva and is refusing to talk.

ii. A 10-year-old boy presents with a persistent dry cough, which is worse at night and while playing at school. He is on steroid cream for eczema but has no other medical history of note.

iii. A 3-year-old girl attends with her mother. She has recently been off her food and has had a mild fever. Her voice has become hoarse and she is constantly coughing in the evenings. Her mother describes the cough as barking.

SBAs

Question 1

A 6-year-old boy is rushed into the ED with suspected meningitis. He is bradycardic, febrile and hypertensive. He has fluctuating levels of consciousness. What should be avoided?

1. Intravenous antibiotics
2. Intravenous fluids
3. Intravenous paracetamol
4. Intravenous steroids
5. Lumbar puncture

Question 2

Which of the following clinical features is not associated with viral gastroenteritis?

1. Diarrhoea
2. Fatigue
3. Fever
4. Poor oral intake
5. Vomiting bile

Question 3

A 10-year-old boy attends with his mother. He has been complaining of intense itching over his hands. On examination the skin is excoriated and there are patches of crusted lesions. His mother explains that his little sister is also developing similar symptoms. Which of the following is the most likely diagnosis?

1. Chickenpox
2. Eczema
3. Hand, foot and mouth disease
4. Impetigo
5. Scabies

Question 4

A 12-year-old girl attends the ED with her aunt. She has noted an offensive green vaginal discharge over the last few days. She is otherwise systemically well with some minor bruises on her upper arm. Which of the following is the most likely diagnosis?

1. Foreign body
2. Immune thrombocytopenic purpura
3. Menstruation
4. Sexually transmitted infection
5. Urinary tract infection

Answers

EMQ ANSWERS

Answer 1

i. **(5) Lobar pneumonia.** The presence of fever, tachypnoea, productive cough and chest signs make pneumonia the most likely diagnosis. The presence of neck stiffness is due to the upper lobe infection. It is important to always rule out meningitis by performing a full examination.

ii. **(8) Menstruation.** It can be alarming for both girls and their parents at the time of menarche, and it is common for them to seek medical advice during the first menstruation.

iii. **(7) Meningococcal meningitis with septicaemia.** It is always essential to rule out meningitis in children who present in this manner. He has photophobia, indicating meningitis, and some clinical features of shock – poor urinary output, drowsiness. A rash is noted and this can quickly spread – this is indicative of meningococcal sepsis. It is essential that the administration of IV antibiotics is not delayed as meningococcal infection can kill in hours.

Answer 2

i. **(4) Foreign body.** It is very common for toddlers to put toys into their mouth. This young girl has no other systemic symptoms, other than a dry cough. It is most common for foreign bodies to travel down the right main bronchus. Often metal detectors are used in the ED to detect objects such as coins.

ii. **(2) Bronchiolitis.** This is a common respiratory infection affecting 1- to 9-month-olds and is usually caused by the respiratory syncytial virus (RSV). Coryzal symptoms often precede breathlessness and a dry cough.

iii. **(1) Appendicitis.** Pain often starts around the umbilicus and then moves to the right iliac fossa. On examination of her abdomen, it is likely that there will be guarding as she is finding it difficult to move and cough. An urgent surgical review should be requested, as she will most likely need to go to theatre for appendicectomy.

Answer 3

i. **(6) Epiglottitis.** This is a life-threatening emergency and urgent assistance should be sought from a senior ENT surgeon and anaesthetist. The patient has a fever, and is unable to swallow or talk. IV antibiotics should only be given after the airway is secure as venepuncture/cannulation can unnecessarily alarm the child and precipitate total airway obstruction.

ii. **(1) Asthma.** Asthma is a clinical diagnosis and is suggested by a history of persistent cough, wheeze and breathlessness, which is worse on exertion. This patient also has eczema which, alongside asthma and allergic rhinitis (hay fever), suggests a history of atopy.

iii. **(3) Croup.** Croup, or laryngotracheobronchitis, is most commonly caused by parainfluenza virus and in children, is the most common cause of acute stridor. Systemic upset may be present with a mild fever. A barking cough is typical of croup. Some children may need admission for further treatment.

SBA ANSWERS

Answer 1

(5) **Lumbar puncture.** Never perform a lumbar puncture in these circumstances. There are possible signs of raised intracranial pressure: hypertension, relative bradycardia and fluctuating consciousness. A lumbar puncture can result in coning of the brainstem through the foramen magnum and should never be performed when there are features of raised intracranial pressure. Performing a lumbar puncture is not a priority as the diagnosis is clear. In this situation there should be no delay in administering IV antibiotics and stabilizing the patient first.

Answer 2

(5) **Vomiting bile.** Vomiting bile, severe abdominal pain and bloody diarrhoea are not features of viral gastroenteritis. If these are present, an alternative cause should be sought such as bowel obstruction.

Answer 3

(5) **Scabies.** It can often be difficult to identify the characteristic appearance of burrows due to secondary infection caused by scratching. The fact that the itching is very intense and that his sister is also developing similar symptoms makes it unlikely to be eczema. The whole family should be treated.

Answer 4

(4) **Sexually transmitted infection.** It is unusual for a 12-year-old to have offensive green vaginal discharge. It is important to rule out sexual abuse as 12-year-olds are unable to have consensual sexual intercourse and this is classed as rape. She also has 'minor' bruises on her upper arms, which may be finger marks or old injuries from other physical abuse. She will need to be admitted so that further investigation can take place and also in order to ensure the child's safety.

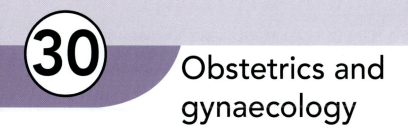

Obstetrics and gynaecology

Questions

EMQs

For each of the questions, select the most likely option from the list of diagnostic options. Answers can be used once, more than once or not at all.

Diagnostic options

1. Appendicitis
2. Dysmenorrhoea
3. Ectopic pregnancy
4. Endometriosis
5. Pelvic inflammatory disease
6. Placenta praevia
7. Polycystic ovarian disease
8. Pyelonephritis
9. Threatened miscarriage
10. Urinary tract infection

Question 1

i. A 25-year-old female presents with worsening sharp right lower abdominal pain and light vaginal bleeding. She has no other medical history of note, other than a treated *Chlamydia trachomatis* infection 3 years ago.

ii. A 16-year-old female presents to the ED with lower abdominal cramps that have been increasing over the last 24 h, during which she has started bleeding vaginally. A urinary pregnancy test is negative.

iii. A 35-year-old female is 30 weeks pregnant with her fifth child. She is concerned, as she has noticed some vaginal bleeding during the day. She has not had any abdominal pain and examination of her abdomen is otherwise unremarkable.

Diagnostic options

1. Appendicitis
2. Ectopic pregnancy
3. Endometriosis
4. Molar pregnancy
5. Pelvic inflammatory disease
6. Placental abruption
7. Pre-eclampsia
8. Pyelonephritis
9. Threatened miscarriage
10. Urinary tract infection

Question 2

i. A 28-year-old female is 35 weeks pregnant with twins. It is her first pregnancy. She is brought to the ED complaining of headache, abdominal pain and nausea. Her husband tells you that she is becoming increasingly confused. Her BP is 165/105.

ii. A 32-year-old female who is 20 weeks pregnant attends with a 2-day history of aching lower abdominal pain. Her BP is 125/75 and a urine dip reveals nitrites.

iii. An 18-year-old female presents with sharp right lower abdominal pain, and she is feeling nauseated. Tenderness is also elicited in the right lower abdomen when pressing the left. She is unable to provide a urine sample for a pregnancy test as she is in too much pain.

SBAs

Question 1

When is anti-D immunoglobulin not needed in rhesus-negative patients?

1. Ectopic pregnancy
2. Miscarriage
3. Normal delivery
4. Placental abruption
5. Speculum examination

Question 2

A 36-week pregnant woman attends with vaginal bleeding. She has previously had three normal vaginal deliveries. History reveals that a recent ultrasound scan indicated a possible low-lying placenta. What should be avoided?

1. Anti-D immunoglobulin if rhesus negative
2. Blood transfusion
3. Examine the abdomen
4. Commencement of intravenous fluids
5. Vaginal examination to assess if labour has started

Question 3

Which of the following clinical features are not associated with pre-eclampsia?

1. Confusion
2. Diplopia
3. Headache
4. Muscle weakness
5. Seizures

Question 4

A 35-year-old woman who is 25 weeks pregnant attends with her partner.
Over the last week she has become increasingly breathless. She was a previous
injecting drug user and is still smoking throughout her pregnancy. She has
a non-productive cough and mild chest pain upon coughing. Which of the
following is the most likely diagnosis?

1. Infective endocarditis
2. Pericarditis
3. Pneumonia
4. Pre-eclampsia
5. Pulmonary embolism

Answers

EMQ ANSWERS

Answer 1

i. **(3) Ectopic pregnancy.** All fertile females presenting with abdominal
pain have ectopic pregnancies until proven otherwise. Always perform
a pregnancy test! Urgent gynaecology review is necessary as deterioration
can occur very rapidly and the patient may need to be taken to theatre
immediately. The previous *Chlamydia trachomatis* infection 3 years ago
suggests that there is likely to be some tubal damage predisposing her to
an ectopic pregnancy.

ii. **(2) Dysmenorrhoea.** Dysmenorrhoea and menorrhagia are common at
the onset of menarche. A negative pregnancy test rules out an ectopic
pregnancy or miscarriage. A full history should be obtained as to when
the pain developed. It is important not to miss other pathology such as
a possible appendicitis. The vaginal bleeding is her period and may be
coincidental with the pain.

iii. **(6) Placenta praevia.** This is more common in females with a high parity.
Vaginal bleeding is often painless although often there may be abdominal
cramps. A vaginal examination should never be performed and an urgent
obstetric opinion should be obtained as there may be compromise to the
foetus. Threatened miscarriage is not an option as this terminology is only
used before 24 weeks gestation.

Answer 2

i. **(7) Pre-eclampsia.** Multiple pregnancies are a risk factor for pre-eclampsia.
Abdominal pain, headache, nausea, confusion and hypertension are
all clinical features of pre-eclampsia. Urine should always be tested for

proteinuria as this makes pre-eclampsia more likely. The obstetric team should assess the patient immediately as complications of pre-eclampsia can often develop. Eclampsia can rarely occur up to a week after delivery as well.

ii. **(10) Urinary tract infection.** Urinary tract infections are more common in pregnancy and should always be treated as they can result in pre-term labour. Always consult the BNF when prescribing for pregnant females.

iii. **(1) Appendicitis.** It is often difficult to obtain urine samples from patients who are in severe pain. Serum β-hCG can be measured to exclude pregnancy as an ectopic pregnancy should always be a differential in any fertile female presenting with abdominal pain. Pain present over the right iliac fossa when the left iliac fossa is palpated is described as Rovsing sign. It is positive in patients with possible appendicitis. A surgical opinion should be obtained and the patient should be fasted and given intravenous fluids.

SBA ANSWERS

Answer 1

(5) **Speculum examination.** Anti-D immunoglobulin should always be given in any situation which risks exposure to rhesus-positive blood in a rhesus-negative patient. This will prevent the formation of antibodies which can occur in future pregnancies. A speculum examination would not result in sensitization.

Answer 2

(5) **Vaginal examination to assess if labour has started.** Never perform a vaginal examination in placenta praevia as this can further precipitate bleeding and cause compromise to the foetus. The other options are all reasonable. An obstetric review should be sought immediately.

Answer 3

(4) **Muscle weakness.** This is not a common feature of pre-eclampsia. Generalized weakness and fatigue can occur, but specific muscle group weakness is unlikely. Always seek expert obstetric opinion immediately in any patient with possible pre-eclampsia.

Answer 4

(5) **Pulmonary embolism.** It is important to realize that medical conditions can also affect pregnancy. Only 50% of DVTs are clinically detectable. This patient has risk factors for a DVT or PE: pregnancy and intravenous drug use. Warfarin is teratogenic in pregnancy and should be avoided. Low molecular weight heparin will need to be initiated after confirmation.

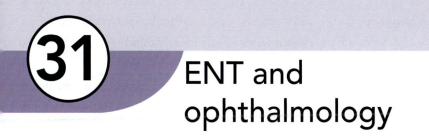

Questions

EMQs

For each of the questions, select the most likely option from the list of diagnostic options. Answers can be used once, more than once or not at all.

Diagnostic options

1. Adenovirus
2. Cholesteatoma
3. Epstein-Barr virus
4. Foreign body
5. Herpes simplex virus
6. *Neisseria gonorrhoea*
7. Rhinovirus
8. *Staphylococcus aureus*
9. *Streptococcus pneumoniae*
10. *Streptococcus pyogenes*

Question 1

i. A 25-year-old male presents with a persistent tonsillitis lasting 3 weeks. He is finding it difficult to swallow and his voice is muffled. He is feeling tired and on examination a mass in the left hypochondrium is also noted.

ii. A 10-year-old male presents with a painful left ear. There is no ear discharge. He is requiring regular analgesia. His mother reports that he ignores her when she is talking to him.

iii. A 35-year-old female presents with a painful left ear. She is complaining of some deafness and itching in her ear. She is otherwise fit and well and is a keen swimmer.

Diagnostic options

1. Acute keratitis
2. Cholesteatoma
3. Conjunctivitis
4. Epstein-Barr virus
5. Foreign body
6. Nasal polyp
7. Otitis externa
8. Orbital cellulitis
9. Preseptal cellulitis
10. Sinusitis

Question 2

i. A 5-year-old male presents with a 3-day history of intermittent epistaxis and foul-smelling discharge from his right nostril.

ii. A 40-year-old female attends the ED complaining of severe right eye pain. Her right eye is red and she dislikes light being shone into this eye. She has no other medical history of note other than asthma and being a contact lens user.

iii. A 30-year-old builder attends with a red left eye. The eye is watering profusely and he is finding it difficult to blink. There is no change in his visual acuity.

SBAs

Question 1

A 38-year-old female presents with unilateral weakness of the right side of her face. On examination she has incomplete eye closure, weakness of her forehead, and vesicles are present within her ear canal. What would not be part of the management of this condition?

1. Aciclovir
2. ENT follow-up
3. Eye lubrication
4. High-dose steroids
5. Topical antibiotic ear drops

Question 2

A 20-year-old female attends with a 3-day history of a worsening sore throat, fever and malaise. On examination, both tonsils are enlarged, erythematous and with exudate. She has cervical lymphadenopathy. What should be avoided?

1. Amoxicillin
2. Difflam® local anaesthetic spray
3. Erythromycin
4. Ibuprofen
5. Penicillin V

Question 3

Which of the following clinical features is not associated with temporal arteritis?

1. Headache
2. Floaters
3. Muscle pain around the shoulders
4. Pain on chewing
5. Vision loss

Question 4

A 75-year-old woman presents with nausea and reduced vision in her right eye which is red and intensely painful, for which she has required morphine. She has a past medical history of hypertension and wears glasses for reading.

1. Acute closed-angle glaucoma
2. Episcleritis
3. Optic neuritis
4. Orbital cellulitis
5. Retinal detachment

Answers

EMQ ANSWERS

Question 1

i. **(3) Epstein-Barr virus.** Glandular fever caused by Epstein-Barr virus can result in a persistent sore throat and general malaise. Hepatosplenomegaly can also result and contact sports should thus be avoided for 3 months.

ii. **(9) *Streptococcus pneumoniae*.** Most cases of acute otitis media are due to *Streptococcus pneumoniae*. Children will present with an acutely painful ear with deafness. The patient's mother reports that her son is 'ignoring' her when she talks to him, which suggests hearing impairment.

iii. **(7) Otitis externa.** This patient has two risk factors with swimming and itching of her ear that predispose her to developing otitis externa. She may need microsuctioning of her ear canal to remove discharge and debris and insertion of an ear wick with topical antibiotic ear drops such as gentamicin.

Question 2

i. **(5) Foreign body.** Children are prone to putting toys and other objects into their noses, ears and mouths. This nasal foreign body has probably been present for a few days as there is now a foul-smelling discharge. This will need removing, and if there is poor compliance from the child, a general anaesthetic may be required.

ii. **(1) Acute keratitis.** Acute keratitis is an acute inflammation of the cornea. Poor contact lens hygiene is a risk factor. This patient will need urgent ophthalmology referral to check for possible ulcers. Steroid drops should not be given.

iii. **(5) Foreign body.** Given this patient's occupation, he is at risk of foreign bodies entering his eye if no eye protection is worn. He will need local anaesthetic drops and a slit lamp examination. Both eyelids should be everted and any foreign bodies carefully removed. Fluorescein should be used to assess his eye for any corneal damage.

SBA ANSWERS

Answer 1

(5) **Topical ear drops.** This patient has a right-side facial palsy. The most likely cause is Ramsay Hunt syndrome, as there are vesicles present in the ear canal. Both aciclovir and a high-dose oral steroid course should be given as well as lubricating eye drops. There is no indication for topical antibiotic ear drops, as the cause is viral in origin.

Answer 2

(1) **Amoxicillin.** Amoxicillin should be avoided as if the sore throat is secondary to Epstein-Barr virus, a widespread maculopapular rash can result. All the other medications can be given safely. Difflam is often helpful in easing painful swallowing.

Answer 3

(2) **Floaters.** Temporal arteritis is commonly associated with polymyalgia rheumatica, which can cause muscle ache and fatigue. Temporal arteritis can cause pain on chewing, pain when combing hair and will result in a raised ESR. The temporal arteries are usually tender to palpation. Floaters are common in a retinal detachment.

Answer 4

(1) **Acute closed-angle glaucoma.** This can typically cause a severely painful, red eye with reduced vision as well as nausea and headache. She will need emergency ophthalmology review, analgesia, antiemetics and miotic drops to reduce the intraocular pressure.

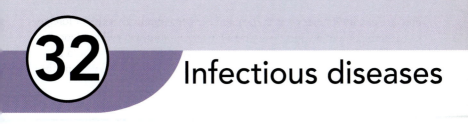

Questions

EMQs

For each of the questions, select the most likely option from the list below.
Answers can be used once, more than once or not at all.

Stem 1 Diagnostic options

1. Cellulitis
2. Gastroenteritis
3. Infective endocarditis
4. Lower urinary tract infection
5. Meningitis
6. Meningococcal septicaemia
7. Necrotizing fasciitis
8. Pericarditis
9. Pneumonia
10. Upper urinary tract infection

Question 1

A 32-year-old male presents to the ED feeling tired and unwell. He is a heroin
user. He is tachycardic and has a temperature of 38°C. On examination you
hear a loud pansystolic murmur at the left sternal edge. His blood tests show a
raised CRP.

Question 2

A 17-year-old male presents to the ED with nausea and headache. He is
normally fit and well, but has been unwell with flu-like symptoms over the
past 24 h. Nobody else in his family is unwell and he has not travelled recently.
He has a temperature of 38.5°C, a heart rate of 85 bpm and blood pressure of
110/80. On examination, he is lethargic and irritable and has a positive Kernig
sign. He has no skin changes or rashes.

Question 3

A 42-year-old woman with poorly controlled diabetes presents to the ED
feeling unwell. She complains of fevers and chills, but has no other symptoms.
She has a temperature of 37.5°C, a heart rate of 80 bpm and a blood

pressure of 140/90. Her chest is clear and her urine dipstick result is normal. On examination of her foot, you find a large area of warm, erythematous skin around her right heel.

Stem 2 Diagnostic options

Which of these investigations would best allow diagnosis in the following situations? Answers may be used once, more than once or not at all.

1. Blood cultures
2. Chest X-ray
3. CT scan
4. ECG
5. Echocardiogram
6. Full blood count
7. Lumbar puncture
8. Skin swabs
9. Urine dipstick
10. Urine microscopy, culture and sensitivity

Question 4

A 19-year-old female presents to ED with fever. She also complains of dysuria and her mid-stream urine shows haematuria.

Question 5

A 50-year-old male presents to the ED with fever and night sweats, which began 3 days ago. He has a prosthetic mitral valve, but is normally well. On examination, he has a temperature of 38.5°C, a heart rate of 105 bpm and a loud pansystolic murmur, which can be heard in all four heart areas.

Question 6

A 20-year-old female who has recently started at university presents to the ED with decreased consciousness. She has a fever of 39°C, a pulse of 110 bpm, a blood pressure of 80/60 and a petaechial rash is developing.

SBAs

Question 1

What are the two most common bacterial causes of cellulitis?
1. *Pseudomonas* and *Streptococcus pyogenes*
2. *Streptococcus pyogenes* and *Staphylococcus aureus*
3. *Streptococcus pneumoniae* and *Staphylococcus aureus*
4. *Staphylococcus aureus* and *Pseudomonas*
5. *Pseudomonas* and *Streptococcus pneumoniae*

Question 2

You are called to see a young man who has recently been involved in a road traffic accident. He was largely uninjured, apart from a graze on his right leg.

The area surrounding the graze is red and hot. You draw around the area and return 10 min later. The patient looks very unwell, the affected area has now spread several centimetres beyond the line you drew and the skin has taken on a blueish hue. What is the most likely diagnosis?

1. Abscess
2. Cellulitis
3. Deep vein thrombosis
4. Myonecrosis
5. Necrotizing fasciitis
6. Scalded skin syndrome

Answers

EMQ ANSWERS

Answer 1

(3) **Infective endocarditis.** A presentation of fever with a new-onset regurgitant murmur is highly suspicious of infective endocarditis. Intravenous drug use, fever >38.0° and an elevated CRP are all suggestive of this also. Echocardiography should be performed, along with blood cultures – three sets over a 24 h period from different sites. A negative result from transthoracic ECHO does not exclude infective endocarditis, and transoesophageal ECHO should be considered if this is the case.

Answer 2

(5) **Meningitis.** Meningitis may present in the classical way with photophobia and neck stiffness, but often its onset is very non-specific. A flu-like prodrome is common. Any patient with high fever and headache should be investigated for meningitis. This young man exhibits other common features including lethargy and the pathognomonic Kernig sign. With no rash or signs of haemodynamic compromise, it is likely that this case is pure meningitis and not septicaemia.

Answer 3

(1) **Cellulitis.** In a patient with fever of unknown aetiology, it is important to rule out common infections such as UTI and pneumonia. In a diabetic patient, especially one with poorly controlled disease, a foot examination is also important as sensation may be dramatically reduced, preventing the patient from noticing the site of infection. Cellulitis commonly presents with warm, red, swollen skin, but may produce symptoms of systemic infection when severe.

Answer 4

(10) Urine microscopy, culture and sensitivity. This patient has presented with typical symptoms of a lower UTI. The quickest and easiest test for this is a bedside urine dipstick test; however this is not as accurate as direct microscopy and culture and does not provide you with the sensitivity of the infecting organism to antibiotics. It is therefore most useful to send a sample of urine for MC&S.

Answer 5

(5) Echocardiogram. High fever, night sweats and a changing murmur in a patient with a prosthetic valve necessitate investigation for infective endocarditis. The most important test for this is an echocardiogram, although blood cultures would also be important.

Answer 6

(1) Blood cultures. The most important diagnosis to rule out in a young person is meningococcal septicaemia. New university students are at particularly high risk of this condition, which presents with decreased consciousness and haemodynamic compromise. The classic non-blanching rash is a late sign. Blood cultures are diagnostic. Lumbar puncture should be avoided in systemic sepsis as there is a risk of introducing infection into the central nervous system. CT scanning of the head should also be considered given the decreased consciousness, although this is unlikely to give the diagnosis.

SBA ANSWERS

Answer 1

(2) *Streptococcus pyogenes* and *Staphylococcus aureus*. Any of the bacteria listed can cause cellulitis, but these two are the most common in both immunocompetent and immunodeficient individuals. *S. pneumoniae* and *Pseudomonas* are important causes of cellulitis in immunocompromised individuals. *S. pneumoniae* often causes a severe, bullous form of the condition.

Answer 2

(5) Necrotizing fasciitis. Necrotizing fasciitis is quickly recognizable as rapidly spreading erythema and oedema. Initially, it may appear similar to cellulitis – red and erythematous. As it progresses, skin becomes blue and black due to thrombosis and necrosis. A key precipitant is trauma to the skin and soft tissues.

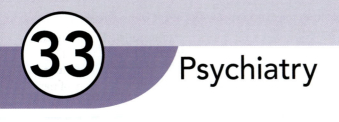

Psychiatry

Questions

EMQs

For each of the following questions, please choose the single most likely condition responsible for the presenting conditions. Each option may be used once, more than once or not at all.

Diagnostic options

1. Acute alcohol intoxication
2. Benzodiazepine overdose
3. Delirium tremens
4. Early alcohol withdrawal
5. Intracranial haematoma
6. Korsakoff's psychosis
7. Opiate overdose
8. Salicylate overdose
9. Tricyclic antidepressant overdose
10. Wernicke's encephalopathy

Question 1

i. A 23-year-old woman collapses outside a nightclub and on examination has pinpoint pupils and bradypnoea.

ii. A 46-year-old man is arrested for drunk and disorderly behaviour. After spending the night in a police cell, a policeman observes him to be sweating and anxious.

iii. A 45-year-old woman with a 5-year history of depression is brought to the ED by her husband, who is concerned that she is not behaving normally. She is confused and on examination, her pupils are dilated.

SBAs

Question 1

A 64-year-old man waiting to be assessed in the ED becomes verbally abusive towards the nursing staff while they try to record their observations. He starts to shout, which the other patients can hear, and there is concern his behaviour may become violent. In the management of a patient with aggression, which of the following is correct?

1. A patient can only be sedated under the Mental Health Act.
2. Manage the aggression before investigating for an underlying cause.
3. Never try to reason with a patient without senior help.
4. The patient will also have clouding of consciousness and therefore should be treated as delirious.
5. The safer route to sedate a patient and defuse the situation is always IV.

Question 2

A 38-year-old woman who has been on lithium for the past 10 years is brought to the ED by her concerned husband. She is normally well controlled on this medication but has had a recent episode of diarrhoea and vomiting. She has a tremor, increased urinary frequency and poor concentration. In suspected lithium toxicity, which one of the following is correct?

1. Check U&Es and TFTs only if the patient has late signs of toxicity.
2. Encourage intake of oral fluids.
3. Reduce medication dose and reassure patient.
4. Stop the drug, get IV access and start a saline drip.
5. Tremor, urinary frequency and poor concentration are late signs of toxicity.

Question 3

A 28-year-old man is found unconscious in his flat. On examination of his eyes, pupils are typical of opioid overdose and there are visible track marks in both antecubital fossae. Which one of the following is correct in opioid overdose?

1. An ABG will show a pattern of respiratory alkalosis.
2. Avoid fully reversing the opioid in addicts.
3. Encourage the patient to go home once he has regained consciousness.
4. On examination, pupils are fixed and dilated.
5. Reverse the overdose with IV flumazenil.

Question 4

A 35-year-old male with a diagnosis of paranoid schizophrenia has been on antipsychotic therapy for the past few months. He is brought to hospital as his GP suspects a side effect of his medication. Which one of the following is true about extrapyramidal side effects of antipsychotics?

1. They never occur in chronic use of antipsychotics.
2. They occur as a result of over-stimulation of dopamine receptors.
3. They should always be treated as an emergency in ICU.
4. They typically present with arrhythmias.
5. They typically present with rigidity of muscles and posturing.

Answers

EMQ ANSWERS

Answer 1

i. **(7) Opiate overdose.** The age of the patient and the presentation are suggestive of an overdose of opiates following recreational drug use. Pinpoint pupils are classically associated with opiates. There are a few other possible causes of fixed pinpoint pupils—pontine haemorrhage and noxious chemical agents—which are far less common. Therefore opiate overdose should always be in your differential diagnosis. The management is respiratory support followed by gradual reversal of the opiate with naloxone.

ii. **(4) Early alcohol withdrawal.** This man has spent a few hours without alcohol and is now in the first stages of withdrawal. Sweating and anxiety are the first symptoms to manifest. It is imperative to explain the importance of having an alcoholic drink before seeking help through an organized rehabilitation programme. If the patient does not have a drink he is at risk of developing delirium tremens, which can be fatal.

iii. **(9) Tricyclic antidepressant overdose.** The history of depression makes TCA overdose most likely. TCAs have a narrow therapeutic index. The dilated pupils are part of the anticholinergic side effects of TCAs. The medication should be stopped and the overdose treated. TCAs are particularly cardiotoxic; therefore continuous ECG monitoring is very important to recognize arrhythmias quickly.

SBA ANSWERS

Answer 1

(2) Manage the aggression before investigating for an underlying cause. An aggressive patient puts you and the patient in a potentially unsafe situation. It is important to ensure safety before continuing with investigation that will require patient contact and invasive methods. The patient with aggression may not have an underlying medical cause; therefore clouding of consciousness does not always apply. It is important to call a senior member of staff to help you in a situation where you are out of your depth. However, a patient may simply only require good communication to diffuse a situation; therefore it is not always essential for senior input immediately. The Mental Health Act is not always appropriate where emergency sedation is required. In that case the patient can be sedated under common law. It may sometimes be necessary to sedate via the intravenous route; however, this is not the safest route as there are more risks associated. If a patient is willing to take oral medication, then always use this approach.

Answer 2

(4) **Stop the drug, get IV access and start a saline drip.** Lithium toxicity is potentially life threatening, requiring immediate management. It is important to stop the drug and assist the body's removal via a saline drip. Late signs of toxicity are confusion, a coarse tremor and ophthalmoplegia. Blood tests should be performed in all patients on lithium who have symptoms, particularly to check renal and thyroid function, which are affected in lithium toxicity.

Answer 3

(2) **Avoid fully reversing the opioid in addicts.** Naloxone is the antidote for opioids and flumazenil is used in some cases of benzodiazepine overdose. Naloxone acts quickly and if the opioid is reversed rapidly, these patients can insist on leaving quickly and are still at risk of further complications. They can also become violent because they have lost their desired effect of the opioid. It is therefore best to reverse the drug gradually if possible. A typical ABG shows a pattern of respiratory acidosis as the patient has respiratory depression. On examination, the patient has pinpoint pupils. There are few other causes of bilaterally constricted pupils. A patient should never be discharged as soon as they regain consciousness from their overdose. Unconsciousness can recur when naloxone wears off and further respiratory depression may occur over the next 6 h; therefore the patient should be observed carefully.

Answer 4

(5) **They typically present with rigidity of muscles and posturing.** Extrapyramidal side effects occur due to their antidopaminergic effect on the basal ganglia. They do not always require emergency treatment and only transfer to ICU if muscles of ventilation are affected or emergency blood pressure control is required. Some side effects are more common after prolonged use, for example akathisia. Some of the side effects can occur after withdrawal or reintroduction of an antipsychotic. Arrhythmias can occur but are not typical; however, it is important to obtain an ECG.

Index